THE AIDS CRISIS IS RIDICULOUS

and Other Writings, 1986–2003

THE AIDS CRISIS IS RIDICULOUS

and Other Writings, 1986–2003

GREGG BORDOWITZ
edited by James Meyer
with a foreword by Douglas Crimp

The MIT Press
Cambridge, Massachusetts
London, England

First MIT Press paperback edition, 2006

This book was set in Adobe Minion MM by Graphic Composition, Inc.

Library of Congress Cataloging-in-Publication Data

Bordowitz, Gregg
The AIDS crisis is ridiculous and other writings : 1986–2003 / Gregg Bordowitz ; edited by James Meyer, with a foreword by Douglas Crimp.
p. cm.
Includes bibliographical references and index.
ISBN 978-0-262-02570-7 (hc : alk. paper), 978-0-262-52459-9 (pb)
1. AIDS (Disease). 2. AIDS (Disease) in art. I. Title.

RC606.55.B67A5 2004
362.196'9792—dc22

2004040154

This book was written for
those who are gone
and others who remain.

CONTENTS

ILLUSTRATIONS

FOREWORD

Douglas Crimp

I think it was my forty-fifth birthday and Gregg's twenty-fifth. In fact, we don't share exactly the same birthday. Gregg's is August 14th, and mine is the 19th. But they're close enough together that we often celebrate them together. That year—it would have been 1989—we celebrated at a Times Square–area gay bar called La Escuelita, "the little school." La Escuelita was then an old-style Latino bar very different from other gay bars I knew.

It was laid out like a forties nightclub, with tables on two sides of a relatively small dance floor. The tables closest to the dance floor—not those against the wall, but those on the spacious side of the room by the two bars—were permanently reserved for regular patrons, who came every Saturday night, bringing with them their own bottles of liquor and ordering only mixers from the bar. It was a cross-gender crowd in all senses that that expression might connote. Most important, unlike most other New York gay bars at the time, there were both men and women. There were butch-femme dyke couples and even visibly gender-coded male couples, usually more daddy-boy than butch-femme or top-bottom. But daddy-boy has too much the connotation of a fetish thing; these were simply couples consisting of an older and a younger guy, with the younger one appearing to be "taken care of" by the older, although the older man was likely getting taken care of too. There was something very sweet, even innocent seeming, about the whole setup, a bit belied by the fact that you had to be frisked for weapons to get into the place. I always assumed it wasn't because they were expecting criminal types, but because the couples I just described were prone to jealousies passionate enough to erupt into violence, so you didn't want any knives or guns around when that happened. This added to the allure of the place for me, I guess because I fantasized luring one of the attractive boys away from his *papi,* something that in spite of occasional flirtations never happened.

La Escuelita had the best Latin drag show in town. It always went on promptly at 1:00 A.M., signaled by the disco version of the opening of Strauss's *Also Sprach Zarathustra.* Latin drag shows meant traditional drag queens pumped full of estrogens and silicone who wore fabulous outfits and lip-synched to the latest soul and disco hits or classics of the genre, like Gloria Gaynor's "I Will Survive," Latin versions of the same, and sometimes boleros by Olga Guillot or La Lupe. La Escuelita was my favorite bar in the eighties. I went there pretty much every Saturday night in the early part of the decade. I knew how to dance the merengue, which I'd learned spontaneously one night at a disco called Star in the Condado in San Juan when a beautiful man who spoke no English motioned to me that he wanted to dance.

There was something about this being my world that made me want to celebrate Gregg's and my birthday there. Something, that is, about wanting to bring Gregg and our ACT UP friends, who were his age, not mine, to my gay scene. Because, you see, I always felt a bit out of place among the ACT UP boys. Funny that an old-style Latin gay bar felt like *my* scene by comparison.

Preparing to write this foreword, I reread Gregg's "My Postmodernism," the essay he wrote for the *Artforum* special issue on the eighties. At the beginning of the piece he recalls, during the period when he was a student at the School of Visual Arts, a "late night at the Pyramid Club on Avenue A in the East Village." I never went to the Pyramid Club in those days, the days when a new kind of ironic drag was being invented, more like performance art than classic drag: John Kelly as Joni Mitchell or the Mona Lisa; Soul Frieda, who had a tiny doll's head for a head; Lypsinka, for whom lip-synching was as much about outré material as impeccable timing. I'm not sure I even knew about the Pyramid Club at that point. I was a West Village fag. Gregg continues about the East Village scene: "The East Village was then host to a hodgepodge of cultures—punk, bohemian, queer, and druggie. No one I knew referred to himself as gay. That identity was reserved for clones—older gay men who wore mustaches and dressed alike in tight jeans and nylon bomber jackets, or in leather." That would have been me, a gay clone, beard, mustache, tight jeans, bomber jacket—the whole package. Illustrating Gregg's *Artforum* essay is a cover of *Outweek* from 1990 featuring "The New Clone vs. the Old Clone," with a picture of our ACT UP friend Peter Bowen styled as the new, East Village clone. I don't recognize the model for the old-style clone. He has a bushy mustache and a bad hairdo. But the contrast in clones is not only a contrast in historical styles, it's a contrast in age. While the new clone is young and sexy, the old clone is over-the-hill. Not only does he still have that dreary old-fashioned look that he had in the seventies, but he dyes his hair and has wrinkles. He probably has AIDS too.

"None of my friends knew much about AIDS in 1986," Gregg writes. "I was still living in a mostly straight-identified scene, and AIDS was a remote concern." But the story Gregg goes on to tell is the one that would bring two generations of gay men, and him and me, together—the story of a growing recognition of our mutual implication in this horrible health crisis and of the necessity to fight the government's criminally neglectful response to it, the story, that is, of ACT UP. Gregg got there before me, right at the beginning, for the first demonstration on Wall Street in March of 1987. I got there because of Gregg. I wanted to publish some material on AIDS in *October,* the journal of which I was an editor. I commissioned Leo Bersani to write a review of Simon Watney's book *Policing Desire,* which became his famous essay "Is the Rectum a Grave?" and I asked my friend Martha Gever to write about Stuart Marshall's 1984 video analysis of AIDS representations, *Bright Eyes.* I'd seen the pilot for the groundbreaking AIDS activist video *Testing the Limits* and heard that Gregg was one of the producing collective's most articulate members, so I contacted him.

Thinking at that point of expanding *October*'s coverage of cultural responses to AIDS to a full-fledged special issue, I asked Gregg about what else we should address. His advice: Go to the ACT UP meetings Monday nights at the Community Center—that's where you'll learn everything you need to know about AIDS issues. It was one of the best pieces of advice I've ever been given, and I don't hesitate to say that following it changed my life. It determined the ultimate shape of the *October* special issue, *AIDS: Cultural Analysis/Cultural Activism,* and it contributed to a shift in my intellectual pursuits in the years that followed, which meant, among other things, leaving *October* and getting a teaching job, as well as expanding my interests beyond contemporary art to cultural studies and queer theory. And it changed my social world, which now increasingly became a world of younger queer artists and intellectuals. Funny, Gregg writes further in "My Postmodernism" of going for the first time in 1986 to the Community Health Project in the Lesbian and Gay Community Services Center in the *West* Village: "On the steps of the center that day, I decided to become a citizen of the gay community." So about the time Gregg found it okay to accept the designation *gay,* I began to discover the utility of the reclaimed term *queer* largely through my friendship with Gregg and his circle.

I'm writing about these crossings of generational identities and their often mutually exclusive spaces of cruising and community in an attempt to suggest something of the disorientation and complexity for me in adjusting to an intellectual friendship with someone half my age and someone whose personal style was so unlike mine, in which I felt as much mentored as mentor (when I published "Mourning and Militancy" in the last issue of *October* I edited, in 1989, I dedicated it to "Gregg Bordowitz, my AIDS activist mentor"). Gregg had all the charisma of a major player in ACT UP—a self-assured speaker to the floor of 300 or 400 fellow activists, an organizer of major actions, and, for that matter, a major crush for maybe half the men and women in the group. I faithfully attended meetings and participated in demonstrations, but I always sat at the side or back of the meeting room and spoke to the floor only once, and I felt extremely self-conscious at demonstrations. I also felt a bit old, a bit out of it, a bit, well, West Village clone among all these vibrant men and women busy reinventing gay activism. Like many members of ACT UP, I admired Gregg and had a bit of a crush on him. And we became friends and intellectual allies. I continued to talk to him about the *October* AIDS issue throughout its long period of production. And he contributed his valuable piece on making *Testing the Limits,* "Picture a Coalition." I'll immodestly admit that, as he generously writes in his introduction to that text, I "taught [him] how to compose an essay." Although that's not quite right. What I think I taught Gregg at that moment is that the essay he was attempting to write tended toward the form of a manifesto, and that he should think of it as such and push it all the further in that direction.

I can't take credit for Gregg's writing style, but I think I recognized it for what it was at that moment and encouraged him to run with it. And I do think Gregg is a fine writer of manifestos. He's a master of the declarative statement. His is an adamantly activist voice. But it's not only that. Certainly Gregg is given to pronouncement, but he's riddled with doubt too. Gregg's greatest achievement, in my estimation, is the wonderful videotape *Fast Trip, Long Drop,* in which Gregg splits himself into two characters, one of whom is, as I wrote in an essay about the work, "funny, sad, lonely, searching, fatalistic. The second is cynical, defiant, furious, dangerous." Interestingly, in the tape it's Alter Allesman, the alter ego, who speaks in pronouncements—"I'm sick and I don't want a cure. I like my illness. . . ." But the absurdity of the statements is a tip-off to the self-doubt and painful self-examination and self-exposure that lies behind them and gets expressed in the video by Gregg's other, "true" self. The real truth, though, is that the true self is both personae, or lies somewhere between the two, or in the constant back and forth from one to the other. What makes this division still more complicated is that these selves are also historical as represented in the tape. There's a younger Gregg making his self-assured activist statements at a demonstration. And then there's the then current Gregg, dressed to appear as that former activist persona montaged into footage from the same demonstration, voicing his doubt, his despair, his utter lack of assurance. It's one of the most brilliant representations of the affective condition of political activism I know of, and one that fully captures my own sense of ambivalence and awkwardness as a participant in movement politics. But the initial activist statement is right too. For Gregg remains extraordinarily ardent in his commitments—political, cultural, intellectual. Gregg's writing and his video production are always carried out in direct, passionate dialogue with the wide range of writers and artists he admires, whether Walter Benjamin or Yvonne Rainer, Charles Ludlam or Janet Flanner.

When I saw *Habit,* Gregg's sequel to *Fast Trip,* I again came up against Gregg's and my differences of generation and identity. The habit of *Habit* is figured largely in terms of Gregg's domestic relationship with Claire Pentecost, or perhaps it is fairer to say that this domestic scene is the *space* of *Habit.* Claire plays a central role in the Chicago part of the tape, but the habit most at issue within this domestic setting is one of daily doses of lifesaving HIV medications together with the humdrum of daily life—doing the laundry, mowing the lawn. Gregg's HIV infection raises painful issues within this scene, issues of his mortality and of Claire's habitual fear that she could lose him.

Between the time that Gregg made *Fast Trip* and *Habit,* I too became infected with HIV, and I also take antiviral medications to safeguard my health. But I have resisted, for a complex of reasons, a domestic relationship, something that I attribute, in less self-reflexive moments, to my adherence to the sexual liberation ethos of my generation of gay men. So for me, a habitual dilemma is disclosing my infection in the context of sexual encounters. Because I think it's most ethical to let my partners decide if they want to have sex with someone who's positive, I am faced with the necessity each time I have sex with someone new of telling him my status. It's either that or no sex. My habitual quandary about sex, HIV infection, and disclosure is entirely unrepresented in *Habit,* in which sex—straight versus gay is *not* the issue here—is only an implied fact of domestically coupled life.

Now, I certainly don't expect to find myself in every representation of AIDS. Especially in a tape that is about the ethical question of privilege in relation to the vast majority of people with AIDS who lack access to life-saving medications, it would be more than a little solipsistic to complain about the lack of attention to my own quotidian troubles. But the fact of *Habit*'s not addressing sex and prevention (which Gregg takes up here in his "More Operative Assumptions") made me aware that Gregg and I currently have very different relations to our HIV infection and how it affects our identities and our senses of the central AIDS issues today. And why wouldn't this be the case? Gregg has been living with HIV for the better part of twenty years, while I've been dealing with it for less than ten. Gregg was diagnosed at a time when AIDS really did seem to be a death sentence; I seroconverted when new antiviral medications held the promise that HIV disease might truly become a "chronic manageable illness." Gregg became infected before AIDS activism began; I, after it was effectively over. Gregg has always written about AIDS as someone living with the disease; most of my writing about AIDS was with the voice of someone uninfected. Gregg's project in *Habit*—like his evolving project in the essays collected here—is thus a very different project from mine in my own collection of AIDS writings, *Melancholia and Moralism.*

Gregg writes about *Habit* here in his "More Operative Assumptions," "The video has a formula, a proposition: the reconciliation of habit and foreignness is intimacy." After a lucid detailing of the function of intimacy in the video, Gregg concludes this part of his discussion with a string of declaratives (distilled from reading Emmanuel Levinas): "Intimacy is an irresolvable dichotomy. One cannot be an 'I' without an Other, yet one can't fully become identical with an Other. Intimacy is a paradox. Being for the Other is an ethical ideal, absolutely necessary, fundamentally inescapable, and ultimately impossible." Reading this, I saw *Habit* differently, more clearly than before. I saw that the South Africa and Chicago portions of the video impinged on each other and enriched each other *because* they remained essentially autonomous. I also understood intimacy more clearly than ever before. Intimacy reconciles but never fully, as Gregg reminds us, the differences that separate us. It makes being in the presence of others possible, even pleasurable, but only if we accept that it will also be difficult, painful. And I understood my friendship with Gregg more clearly than ever before.

Our birthday party at La Escuelita in 1989 was a lot of fun. We danced the merengue, we saw a great drag show. But we've celebrated many better, more intimate ones since.

EDITOR'S NOTE

James Meyer

The AIDS crisis has produced an estimable literature, which has come to be known as AIDS writing. Writing around AIDS records the experiences of AIDS, experiences that verge on the inarticulate and incomprehensible. Much like the fiction of Edmund White, the memoirs of Paul Monette, the confessions of David Wojnarowicz, the plays of Larry Kramer and Tony Kushner, and the poetry of Thom Gunn, the writings of Gregg Bordowitz explore the salient themes of the genre: living with a disease while witnessing the deaths of loved ones and friends; the prejudice that HIV-positive people face; and the ethical questions that AIDS poses, such as the relations of conduct between the sick and well.

And yet within the idiom of AIDS writing Bordowitz's texts assume a place occupied, so far as I know, by no other. The particular stake of this collection is its proposal of a theory of art-making developed in response to an epidemic. *The AIDS Crisis Is Ridiculous* is a testimony of one person's experience of living with HIV; but it is also the record of a *practice,* a practice organized to address a public health crisis. AIDS activist artists quickly learned that the epidemic necessitates a highly pragmatic approach, a capacity to transform the very terms of one's practice. Bordowitz's early work, produced collaboratively within the ambience of ACT UP, contested dominant representations of AIDS and recorded the movement's actions (Bordowitz filmed the very first ACT UP demonstration at the New York Stock Exchange in 1987). His practice then moved into AIDS education, and then to presenting more nuanced images of people living with HIV for people living with HIV. Other videos and texts have addressed aspects of the epidemic in a highly allusive manner.

This book is an account of an artist's practice, but it is not merely this. For Bordowitz writing is itself a practice, a marshaling and combining of different discursive forms. His texts traverse several modes. The first, following the work of Michel Foucault, Eve Kosofsky Sedgwick, Cindy Patton, Simon Watney, and Douglas Crimp, critiques representations of people with AIDS and gays and lesbians, and the political and social institutions that work against their interests; this is the "queer" vein of Bordowitz's project. In the second, formalist mode, the artist's practice becomes an object of reflection. Filmic and video form and issues of spectatorship are foregrounded. Masters of avant-garde cinema and theater, ranging from

Sergei Eisenstein and Bertolt Brecht to Yvonne Rainer, become key references. (The director Charles Ludlam, whose concept of Ridiculous Theater inspired the title essay of this book, occupies a place between the first and second tendencies.)

The third vein of Bordowitz's writings—inspired by psychoanalytic theory and the media studies work of Raymond Williams and Stuart Hall—recognizes television as a dominant force in the contemporary construction of subjectivity. Beginning with "Picture a Coalition," Bordowitz posits a counterpractice centered not on the production of art video but *television,* a television that takes as its ambition a dissolution of the traditional, Greenbergian divide between critical and mass media forms (the artist's Brechtian affiliation is also apparent here). The final, "literary" aspect of Bordowitz's writings—apparent in such texts as "New York Was Yesterday" and "Which Is More Powerful, the Word or the Idea?"—may be understood as a response to activism's ultimately limited grasp of the full range of the epidemic's complexities. An imaginative and philosophical literature—texts by Janet Flanner, J. G. Ballard, Walter Benjamin, Emmanuel Levinas, Nicolai Erdman, and Fyodor Dostoyevsky—are the writer's starting point. The clarion tone of "Picture a Coalition" gives way to confessions of doubt, clear-mindedness to irrationality. Fantasy enters, as well as its converse, the everyday—the space of boredom and habit. The literary enters at the point where the confident discourses of theory and the avant-garde retreat. Much like the finest AIDS writing, Bordowitz's texts in this vein ask questions they cannot answer, questions without answers.

To see Bordowitz's writings as merely an exegesis of his art, a supplement to his video production, is thus to misunderstand their function and importance. Bordowitz's engagement with these discursive traditions suggests that writing is an equal and integral part of his activity. As

Bordowitz's friend and teacher, Craig Owens observes in the essay "Earthwords," a discussion of Robert Smithson's *Collected Writings:*

> The argument which reduces these artists' writings to a secondary, derived position vis-à-vis their work might be diagnosed as one symptom of a modernist aesthetic, specifically, its desire to confine the artist within the sharply delineated boundaries of a single aesthetic discipline. This desire is sanctioned by an unquestioned belief in the absolute *difference* of verbal and visual art.

Owens instead proposes an allegorical notion of practice: art conceived as a palimpsest of media and forms, a semantic overlapping of image and text. Meaning, no longer tied to medium, is destabilized and deferred. "This eruption of language into the aesthetic field . . . ," Owens continues, "is coincident with, if not the definitive index of, the emergence of postmodernism." For Owens, the figure of the artist-writer—the visual artist whose practice traverses language—is paradigmatically postmodernist.

The artist-writer has gone into hibernation since his heyday of the sixties, when Smithson, Rainer, Donald Judd, Robert Morris, Carl Andre, and Sol LeWitt (Owens's exemplars) established writing as a central part of their projects. Today, few younger artists write so audaciously—if they write at all. *The AIDS Crisis Is Ridiculous* is a riposte to this anti-intellectual tendency, which has more or less dominated the American art world since the collapse of postmodernism in the early nineties. With the publication of this book the artist-writer returns. For Bordowitz *is* an artist-writer. As his practice suggests, artists need not be inarticulate, "instinctive" thinkers solely concerned with the orchestration of image, of visual form. To the contrary, *The AIDS Crisis Is Ridiculous* reminds us that artists do have the capacity to develop their ideas within the domain of writing, and writing, so construed, may be counted within the domain of the artistic.

AUTHOR'S NOTE

The texts in this book and all to which they refer are informed by the AIDS crisis. Though I have endeavored to lead a rich intellectual life, and I possess many interests, the threat that the epidemic has posed to me and everyone around me has filtered my thinking. The only text in the book that does not bear the burden of AIDS at all is the first essay, "Geography Notes." Written before my awareness of the disease, it provides a glimpse into the preoccupations that preceded my involvement in the crisis. These concerns were specifically tied to art and aesthetics. They were never abandoned in the work that followed. Rather these interests were given focus and urgency.

There are texts included here that do not directly address AIDS. However, the epidemic animated the ideas from the margins. So total was the burden of illness—mine and others'—that the only viable response, other than to cease making art entirely, was to adjust to the gravity of the predicament by using the crisis as a lens. Indeed, AIDS touches every issue imaginable: sex, love, death, economy, drugs (recreational and medicinal), morals, ethics, representation, and culture.

This collection starts with essays that address formal concerns in a straightforward manner: "Geography Notes," "Picture a Coalition," "The AIDS Crisis Is Ridiculous," and "Operative Assumptions." For the most part I have left the earliest writings in this collection untouched, minimally altering only those formulations I now find insufficient. In some cases I have appended footnotes to add new thoughts to an old text. I wanted to retain both the youthful exuberance and the palpable sense of fear in the writing.

A shift occurs toward the middle of the book. The writing takes on a more experimental character, as the prose itself becomes a subject of the texts: "Boat Trip," "Dense Moments," "Present Tense," and a selection from my columns written for the journal *Documents* titled "New York Was Yesterday." The columns mix fiction and fact. The writing evolves entirely into fiction in "Which Is More Powerful: The Word or the Idea?"

The last third of the volume extends themes that were explored in the beginning. Current events regarding the global AIDS pandemic compelled me to reformulate activist concerns in "What the World Needs Now" and "The Effort to Survive AIDS from the Point of View of a Race-Car Driver." Invited by *Artforum* to revisit the eighties for their fortieth anniversary issue gave me an opportunity to reexamine the underlying ideas of my practice and the history that formed them in "My Postmodernism." Finally, I wrote the concluding essay—"More Operative Assumptions"—specifically for this book, in order to sum up my theoretical concerns as they have developed to the point of this publication.

There is another point of entry into my writing apart from AIDS. From the beginning of my mature practice—the moment "when I found my voice"—I've been engaged by the problems of autobiography. The films of Yvonne Rainer were most influential in this regard. I recall an epiphany watching *The Man Who Envied Women.* I realized that to describe the world around me I had to "cut across" my own subjectivity and submit the "slice" to close scrutiny; kind of like counting the rings of growth on the trunk of a fallen tree. I adopted the method as my own.

Having a disease defines my world, and the disease is a global problem. These are two very different concepts. The first clause describes a subjective condition. The second describes an objective condition. The two clauses can only be bridged through language by using a conjunction. Can the two conditions be joined in the realm of practice? This is no mere exercise. I believe that the key to understanding and fighting the AIDS crisis depends on the conjunction of the subjective experiences of people with AIDS and the objective conditions of the crisis. I have an enormous expectation of prose. I continue to believe that if it can be written then it can be realized.

No writer works alone. I am grateful for the support of many people. First, I would like to thank the editor, James Meyer. I could not imagine working on this collection with any editor other than James Meyer; I trust no one more to edit my writing. Alex Alberro first had the idea for this book. Alex approached James to edit the collection, and together they made the proposal to The MIT Press. Executive Editor Roger Conover and Assistant Editor Lisa Reeve were generous with their understanding, support, and assistance. Thank you to Editor Judy Feldmann and Designer Emily Gutheinz for their work and expertise. I want to thank Douglas Crimp for writing the foreword and for his friendship. Zoe Leonard contributed a number of her photographs to accompany the selections from "New York Was Yesterday." It's a privilege to be able to include them here. The photographs intensify the feelings I wish to evoke with the column and they also mark the presence of a rich and enduring amity between us.

I want to acknowledge all the editors I worked with in the past who helped me shape the previously published material in this volume: Jack Bankowsky, Julia Bryan-Wilson, Melodie Calvert, Barbara Hunt, Esther Kaplan, Miwon Kwon, Don McMahon, Helen Molesworth, Tom Lawson, Pratibha Parmar, Michael Renov, Rodney Sappington, Tyler Stawlings, Erika Suderberg, and Jennifer Terry.

I want to give a special acknowledgment to Lynne Tillman, who has always encouraged my writing. She was a pillar of support while I compiled this book.

Yvonne Rainer continues to be the model artist for me. Thank you for your example and your friendship.

My family always stands by me. Thank you to my parents Linda and Martin Bordowitz; to my grandparents Max and Gloria Glassman; and to my sister Traci. Sadly, my paternal grandparents and both of their children are gone: Helen and Harry Harstein, my father Les, and my aunt Andrea. I wish you were here for this.

I am extremely fortunate to have many interlocutors with whom I continue to share ideas. I want to thank you all: Sam Avrett, David Barr, Jean Carlomusto, Yau Ching, Ron Clark, Moyra Davey, Mark Dion, Dan Eisenberg, Richard Elovich, Steve Fagin, Andrea Fraser, Martha Gever, Faye

Ginsberg, John Greyson, Catherine Gund, Mark Harrington, Jill Harris, Bill Horrigan, Omar Karmi, Steve Kurtz, Ernie Larsen, Sherry Millner, Nadja Millner-Larsen, Jennifer Montgomery, Ulrike Müller, Ray Navarro, Craig Owens, Michael Rooks, Abe Rybeck, Jason Simon, Jeffrey Skoller, Peter Staley, Kendall Thomas, Faith Wilding, and Daniel Wolfe.

Thanks to the therapists I have had over the years: Mr. Hoberman, Louis Fourcher, and Mary Doheny. Many of the insights you led me to are contained within the margins. And thank you to my physicians: Dr. Howard Grossman and Dr. John Phair. Your care helped me to remain alive and well enough to continue working.

Thank you to my colleagues and students at the School of the Art Institute of Chicago and the Whitney Museum Independent Studio Program. I am grateful for the assistance of Andrea Goldman, Megan Rider, and Paige Sarlin who helped me compile the manuscript and illustrations.

Finally, the greatest portion of my gratitude goes to Claire Pentecost. She read all of my writing before publication. We shared everything for ten years. Every word I uttered aloud was for her ear first.

Geography Notes: A Survey

1

Originally published as "Geography Notes," *Real Life Magazine* 16 (autumn 1986): 12–17. Minor revisions have been made for consistency.

THIS WAS THE FIRST SIGNIFICANT ATTEMPT *on my part to fit the work of a peer into a genealogy descended from the older artists we admired. I was living with Andrea Fraser at the time. I watched her rehearse her performance in the character of the museum docent, Jane Castleton, for the exhibition "Damaged Goods" at the New Museum in 1986. The chief preoccupation that Andrea and I shared at the time concerned the notion of a materialist geography. We thought that relations among people and things were spatial and that space itself was a capitalist product. Blending Marxism with the psychoanalytic theory of Jacques Lacan, her practice charted the course of the body's movement through the museum's space—a minefield of associations not necessarily tied to the referents or objects in the exhibition.*

Many of the ideas for this article were produced out of frequent conversations with Mark Dion. Mark and I were in daily contact at the time. Tom Lawson gave me the opportunity to publish this, my first essay, in Real Life Magazine. *I wrote it when I was twenty-two.*

Chapter 1
Geography Notes: A Survey

From where he was standing he couldn't get a clear view.

Joseph Kosuth's installation at the Castelli Gallery, "Zero & Not," exemplifies the now canonical strategies and tactics of conceptual art. The walls are to be read as text—a strategy of literalization that attempts to show the extent to which context affects the meaning of the work of art. We are to infer that signification is the combined effect of context and production.

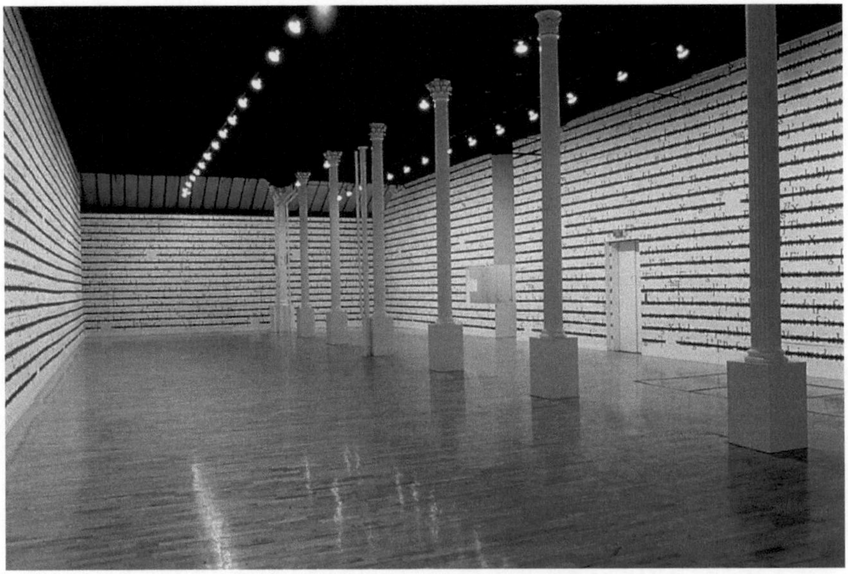

Figure 1.1 Joseph Kosuth, *Zero and Not,* 1986. Joseph Kosuth Leo Castelli Greene Street Gallery, 1986. Courtesy of Joseph Kosuth.

The cancelation of the text, or rather of the wall as text, approximates the operations of erasure objects perform on the viewing space. One has to think about the way paintings obscure the wall, rendering the viewing space apparently neutral, so that the act of viewing seems unmediated, and the conditions for viewing seem natural. This work self-consciously mimics these operations.

The color-coded bars and letters appear to function as ways of knowing, as systems of ordering that normatively form one's understanding of the known.

The text. Although it seems appropriately chosen, it remains inconsequential. The paragraph is culled from a much larger body of psychoanalytic theory to which it cannot sufficiently refer as presented.

The subject of the exhibition is the space for viewing itself. The act of reading is reflexively thrown back onto the viewer. The important point the work makes is that context mediates reading, and thus institutes meaning to such an extent that the work cannot presume a place from which to speak.

Yet Castelli Greene Street is not the only structure that circumscribes meaning around that site. The gallery space is coextensive with much larger systems of organization that are contained within the context of the gallery walls.

The propositions of conceptual art refer only to the artwork's condition of being, in a reflexive way. The conditions of its production, the conditions of its context (outside the gallery walls), and the conditions of its distribution are tacitly ignored. The work remains a benign reaffirmation of the gallery structure's primacy over the conditions of art making.

He shifted his position to get a different view.

Martha Rosler's project stems from similar theoretical conditions that shaped conceptual art. However, implicit in her work is a critique of the formal underpinnings that entrapped conceptual art in academia.

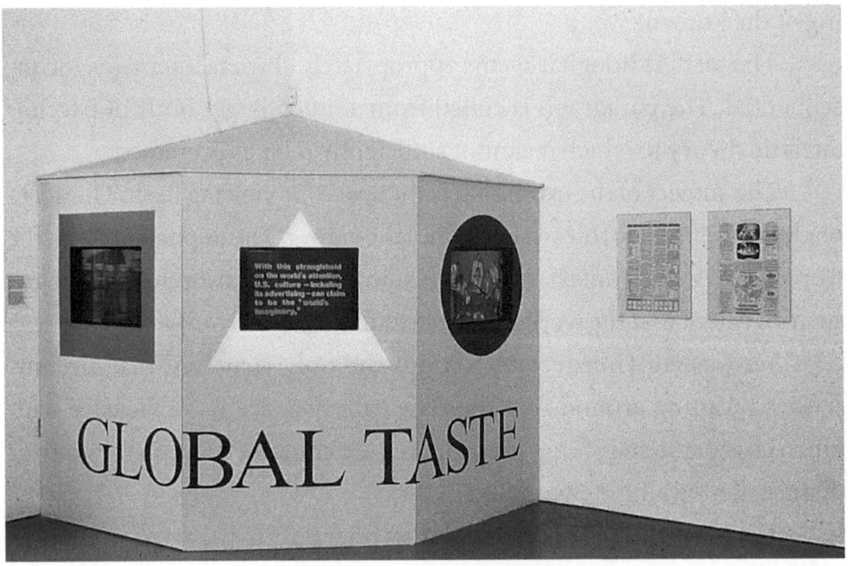
With this stranglehold
on the world's attention,
U.S. culture —including
its advertising—can claim
to be the "world's
imaginary."
GLOBAL TASTE

Figure 1.2 Martha Rosler, *Global Taste: A Meal in Three Courses*, 1985. Courtesy of Martha Rosler.

"The installation, 'Global Taste: A Meal In Three Courses,' has colonization as its theme: colonization of the self and of other countries by media and advertising. The central interlocking motifs in its three videotapes are children, food commercials and learning."[1] But the three video monitors are contained within a structure that makes it impossible to get a view of all at one time. A fragmented collage of material, "Global Taste" pictures the geopolitical relations that form the organizing principles of cultural production. Understanding the art world as a subsidiary of a much larger culture industry, the installation cuts across a miasma of cultural artifacts to make connections between the place of viewing and a view of the world.

The work addresses the increasing homogenization of culture that results from the efforts of the multinational corporations which govern its manufacture.

The installation is an attempt to breach the confines of the viewing condition by way of reference to the disparate forces that compose a world picture.

He turned to see if anyone else was watching.

In a still from Yvonne Rainer's film, *The Man Who Envied Woman,* we see William Raymond as Jack Deller, a middle-aged, successful academic, drink in hand, as he pictures his relation to the world. He stands viewing a collage of material from a number of diverse sources all pinned to the wall. His scrutiny of this stuff suggests one point of view from a position of privilege: male heterosexual, white, educated, liberal left, and relatively affluent. In the film we watch this character order and reorder the bits of

1. Martha Rosler, "Global Taste: A Meal In Three Courses," gallery statement, "The Art of Memory: The Loss of History," The New Museum of Contemporary Art. New York, 1985.

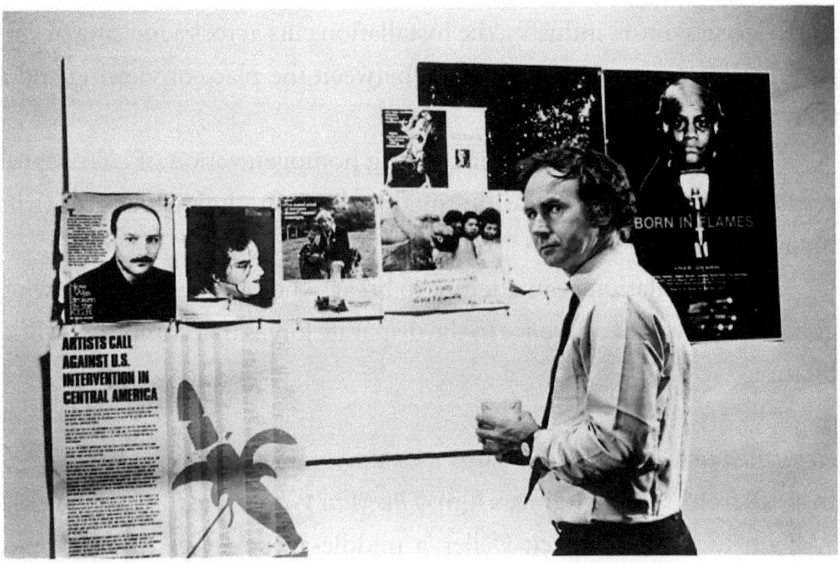

Figure 1.3 Yvonne Rainer, *The Man Who Envied Women,* 1985. Courtesy of Yvonne Rainer.

reportage. He can't find a settling resolution. A fragmented voice-over comments on his activity—readings in different voices, accents, and genders accompany his movements as he shifts the elements of the collage around. The elements reflect an idiosyncratic selection of material out of a general field of concerns—"How I Was Broken by the KGB" from a "*New York Times* Sunday Magazine," a poster from Artists Call Against U.S. Intervention in Central America, an ad for Macanudo cigars, an image of a stressed middle-aged woman from a pharmaceutical ad, a poster for Lizzie Borden's film, *Born In Flames,* and a picture of murdered civilians who are victims of repression by right-wing forces in Guatemala.

The Deller character's presence within the frame and his mimed speculation produce a self-reflexive situation for the viewer of the film. Using the spatial strategies of cinema by juxtaposing image and sound, Rainer gives us a picture of how a worldview is drawn. Deller is a viewing subject being observed by an alternative subjectivity constructed outside the frame of the image through the use of voice-over on the sound track. The filmmaker interrogates a worldview as it is constructed from a position of privilege. Refuting an idealist conception of the singular viewing subject, the situation allows for a number of sexed, class-conscious readings to coincide.

Fast-forward/scan. These loose-ended jottings establish the fundamental principles of a pictorial activity informed by a materialist geography. Mapping is a way of imagining a site in terms of its geographic and historical specificity, as it is viewed through the prism of a fragmented subjectivity.

He walked through the doors and paid the admission fee.

> Hi. My name is Jane Castleton and I'd like to welcome all of you to the New Museum of Contemporary Art. Today, I'll be giving a

> gallery talk for the main, ah, exhibition currently on view; "Damaged Goods: Desire and the Economy of the Object," an exhibition about commodities and consumption, about presentation and display.[2]

Andrea Fraser enters the lobby of the New Museum and claims to be a docent. She then proceeds to deliver a lecture that maps the forces circumscribing the area of the exhibition. The character she assumes is fictional. Its subjectivity is shaped by the same forces that modify the environment of the space. She is the subject viewing/viewed.

> . . . And ah, over here, conveniently located in the bookstore/gift shop, behind this panel is the control board for the museum's security system—owning and exhibiting art, like all valuable property, is a responsibility, and the Museum's first responsibility is to protect the culture it fosters.

The security system was designed by a company appropriately named American Security Systems—"a company that cares as much about aesthetics as it does about protection." Fraser goes on to appraise the placement of the system's features in aesthetic terms, and in particular to discuss their relation to the architectural elements of the space. The parts of the system are rendered coextensively with the architecture—with the order of the space. The system is read as a technology of power that reinforces the boundaries of the area, like a defense-weapons system that seals the perimeters of national boundaries.

At the entrance to the exhibition Fraser/Castelton turns and says:

2. All quotations from Andrea Fraser's event were excerpted from transcripts of the lecture.

> "Damaged Goods: Desire and the Economy of the Object." Now, what is that supposed to mean? Well the phrase, damaged goods, evokes a number of associations for me. It may describe the state of inadequately packaged, or slightly used products. Or, for some it refers to women who aren't virgins. It's also the title of a movie about venereal disease.

Speaking the title of the exhibition, for the second time in the lecture, Fraser takes possession of the title through her voice. She speaks the title in the role of a subject viewing the show. By doing this, Fraser's character articulates a woman's point of view.

She ushers the group toward the women's room, then, standing in front of the door:

> . . . Move in closer—this is a small work and I want all of you to be able to see it . . . This particular image—as those of you who are familiar with so-called international symbols may already know—is supposed to represent a woman. A woman, or rather even women in general, women as such, women as a universally homogeneous category.

Mistaking the international symbol on a toilet door for art is a paradigmatic example of a subject's misrecognition of the image of her body as herself.

> I'd like to resemble a woman. Wouldn't it be nice to resemble a woman?

In this event Fraser uses misrecognition as a strategy for rendering apparent the specular relations implicit in the act of viewing. These relations are not resolved in speculative terms, describing the relation of subject to object. Rather, these relations are transcribed materially, onto Fraser's body.

Misrecognition as a tactic incorporates the fictional condition of signification—the false marriage of sign to referent—into a strategy of truth production. Confusing the objects in front of her for something else, the mediatrix (Fraser as Castleton) forefronts signification as the intermediary agency of the docent. In this way Fraser refers to the conditions of signification within the context of the lecture only to undermine the authority of the pedagogical position she assumes. In doing this she calls into question the enterprises that verify art as art, the criteria of aesthetic judgment.

How does she do this? She mimics the tone of condescension in a grade school teacher's voice. The gestures she makes while addressing the objects at hand are borrowed from Carrol Merril, Vanna White, and a number of other game-show display beauties.

She addresses one of Allan McCollum's *Perfect Vehicles* (confusing it with a porcelain from the Ming Dynasty), and quotes from the Metropolitan Museum of Art guidebook:

> In it is combined the freedom and energy of a newly ripened art form with the sophistication of concept and mastery of execution that comes only with maturity.

Gesture and voice are choreographed to emphasize the artificiality of terms used to attribute high art status to the object. By calling such terms into question, Fraser escapes the self-referential prison of established conceptual art, unable to refer to anything outside the exhibition itself.

> Looking at another *Perfect Vehicle:* This deer-shaped vessel is said to be from Chicama, the valley north of Chan Chan. The deer-shaped vessel has been common to the north of Peru for about two thousand years. During the fourteenth and fifteenth centuries the Chimu Kingdom ruled the north of Peru from its capital at Chan Chan. Its

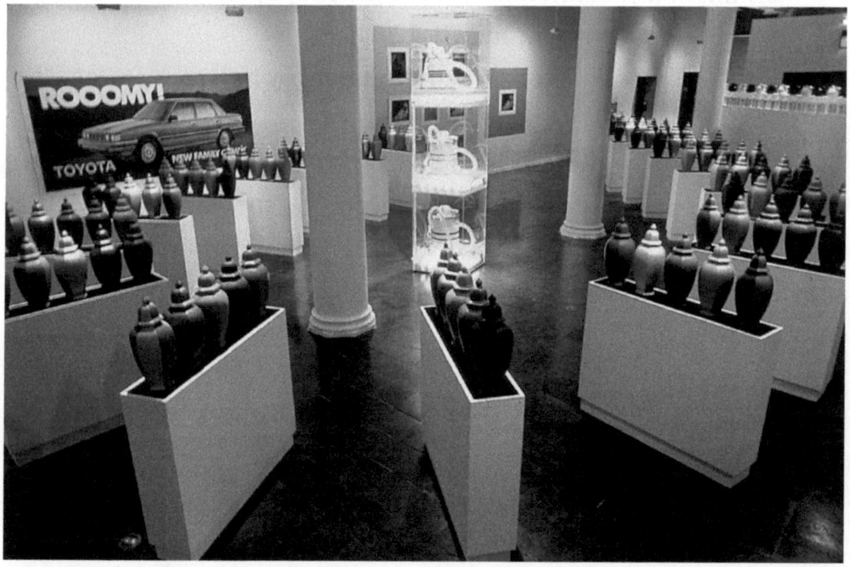

Figure 1.4 Allan McCollum and Jeff Koons, *Damaged Goods,* installation view. New Museum, New York, 1986. Courtesy of the New Museum of Contemporary Art, New York.

monarchs amassed great wealth and constructed enormous walled compounds from which to protect it. These compounds contained so many objects made of precious metals that during Spanish colonial times they were exploited as mines. Current estimates suggest that there may have been about eighty million Native Americans in Latin America when Columbus "discovered" the continent. By 1650, 93percent of this population had been wiped out. The systematic extermination of Latin America's indigenous population continues today in Brazil, Paraguay, and Guatemala.

This vessel was given to the museum by Nelson A. Rockefeller.

She is obviously not talking about *Perfect Vehicles,* or is she? Making use of their appearance as surrogate objects, she attributes an obviously false origin to their making, then associates domination, exploitation, and imperialism as forces identified with the same ruling class that values and owns art. Supplementing McCollum's tactic of mute refusal, Fraser acts against the formalist's limitation of self-referentiality. Standing in the center of the exhibition she says:

> Charles Saatchi, art collector and cofounder of the world's largest advertising firm. It's exciting when Saatchi buys. He's voracious and influential. He buys across the board, and when he buys, the momentum just keeps growing.

Considering the situation of the exhibition in the form of a docent lecture, we learn that it is usually the "product of a certain milieu, of a power structure, of contracts between a corporation and its clients." In telling us this Fraser bares the forces that govern the fabrication of such lectures, and such exhibitions.

Fraser has to use a number of voices and personae to present the collage of material the lecture is composed of. Shifting voices and positions, she presents a number of complex relations; the area marked by the choreography of her movements becomes a site where geopolitical fronts coincide to offer a view of this exhibition, in view of global relations. For example, standing in front of a Jeff Koons poster piece she recounts stories of how Imelda Marcos was duped into buying millions of dollars of art with no real market value. Then, in the voice of a newscaster, tells us that Amnesty International has identified eighty-eight individuals tortured under the Marcos government. Fraser switches voice again, becoming frightened, introspective as she narrates a first-person account of torture. Then, immediately, she is back to the newscaster's monotone.

Throughout the lecture Fraser's presentation is stilted and fragmentary. "Idiosyncratic" is a polite way of describing the schizophrenic syntax of the event. This effectively sets up a speculative relation for the audience, allowing for response according to the spectator's gender, class, or sexuality. A total view is not possible. Glimpses of actualities are presented, affected, as endemic to another viewer's process of cognition. U.S. foreign policy, multinational corporate organization of the world's labor and resources, the arrangement of a single global market—all are laid out within the geography of the exhibition according to the combined effect these forces have in relation to the cartographer and her activity.

A pictorial activity informed by a materialist geography furthers the development of political reflection upon space, and it reveals the spatial strategies of power.[3] These strategies are analyzed in terms of how they form subjectivity, or rather how they coincide with the numerous positions we occupy as social beings. Regarding signifying practices, this

3. Massimo Quaini, *Geography and Marxism* (New York: Barnes and Noble, 1982).

requires an understanding of the spatial configurations of the exhibition space itself. Mapping the geography of this situation necessitates:

[that an anterior space be noted and drawn.

[that a place as defined by the limits of its area can be viewed as separate from the location it is assigned through discourse.

[that the physical boundaries of a space are not limited to the perimeter of a location.

The proposition of this article is this: once the space of exhibition can be pictured in geographic terms, that is, in terms of geopolitical and spatial relations, one can articulate the ways knowledge shapes a view of the world according to the dictates of power.[4]

4. This article and its focus on Andrea Fraser's contribution to *Damaged Goods* shows a preoccupation with the unconscious forces in play for each viewer of an exhibition. Andrea and I were interested in a geography that included the topology of the viewers' psyches. Within the context of art history these interests stem from Surrealism. Freud and Lacan provided the theoretical models for our approach. Recently I have become aware of the writings of psychoanalyst Andre Green, whose ideas concern the "historical perspective" that must be recognized as part of the analytic situation between doctor and patient. Green's "historical perspective" includes:

what has happened,
what has not happened,
what could have happened,
what has happened to someone else but not me,
what could not have happened,
and finally—to summarize all these alternatives about what has happened—a statement that one would not have even dreamed of as a representation of what really happened.

Outside the context of psychoanalysis, this list could be very useful to artists who want to explore the actively present—though not consciously apprehended—

material constituting works of art. By material I mean not only the substance of the work of art itself. I include among the psychic lives of all participating agents captured within the field of the exhibition: artists, curators, preparators, security guards, collectors, and viewers. For more about Green and his "historical perspective" see Andre Green, *Andre Green at the Squiggle Foundation,* edited by Jan Abram (London and New York: Karnac Books, 2002), 2–3.

Picture a Coalition

2

Originally published as "Picture a Coalition," *AIDS: Cultural Analysis, Cultural Activism,* edited by Douglas Crimp (Cambridge: The MIT Press, 1988), 183–196. Minor revisions have been made for consistency.

IN 1987, THE AIDS ACTIVIST MOVEMENT EMERGED *in its most militant form: ACT UP, the AIDS Coalition to Unleash Power. After I attended its first demonstration, I joined the group. Around the same time I co-founded the Testing the Limits video collective. We were very busy running around the five boroughs with video equipment documenting various activist efforts.*

One day, out of the blue, I received a call from Douglas Crimp, then an editor of the prestigious journal October. *I was shocked and intimidated. Of course, I knew who he was; we read his essays in school.* October *was then mandatory reading for serious artists. Douglas heard about my efforts through a mutual friend (Cathy Scott, who worked with Paper Tiger Television) and he invited me to dinner at his house to discuss an issue of* October *entirely devoted to the AIDS crisis. Enthusiastically I told him all about the great work that people were doing to fight AIDS: needle exchanges in the Bronx, prevention efforts in the gay community, treatment initiatives by people with AIDS. Douglas invited me to contribute to the AIDS issue of* October.

The first draft of my essay was a typewritten, single-spaced, five-page screed. Douglas rightly rejected it, kindly, with compassion, and gave me another chance. I returned later with a more coherent version, though it still very much needed editing. Douglas sat with me at the computer in the October *office on Union Square and taught me how to compose an essay.*

This text became the template for a kind of writing that I continue to do today: a theoretical self-analysis that explains in detail the ways that political issues and actions are coextensive with the form of my video work.

Chapter 2
Picture a Coalition

As a twenty-three-year-old faggot, I get no affirmation from my culture. I see issues that affect my life—the issues raised by AIDS—being considered in ways that will probably end my life. For this reason I think that if there is to be a movement that will shift the discussion of AIDS away from the moralizing, punitive attitude that has characterized this country's policy, it will be built out of an emergent popular culture, one that affirms the

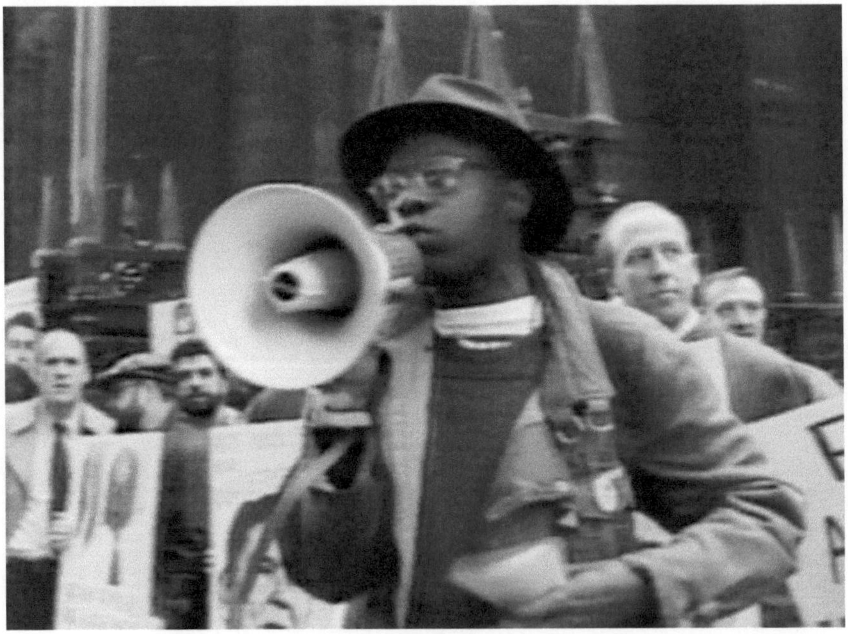

Figure 2.1 *Testing the Limits: New York,* Testing the Limits collective, 1987.

lives of those affected. It will be a counterculture that will grow out of a broad-based mobilization to end the global epidemic.

There are already moves to contain this growing activism. Threats of mass mandatory HIV-antibody testing and quarantine are written in banner headlines. Certain individuals and groups have already been subject to such assaults—within those institutions where surveillance is most easily enforced. This is not even to mention the discrimination people living with AIDS (PLWAs) have faced in all aspects of social life. The first targets of repression are, as always, the most disenfranchised. Thus, New York City's health commissioner Stephen Joseph has recently called for consideration of "mandatory AIDS testing *[sic]* for prostitutes and sex and drug offenders, as well as a heavy crackdown on all forms of prostitution."[1]

What purpose will enforced testing serve? Test results will establish much more than the extent to which a population has been exposed to a virus. Their purpose is to identify an entire social group on the basis of the presence of antibodies. A whole new class of people will be designated as seropositives. The limits of the AIDS community will be established.

1. Ronald Sullivan, "AIDS Test Is Weighed in Sex Cases," *New York Times,* November 21, 1987.

On December 10, 1987, members of the Metropolitan Health Association, an affinity group of gay AIDS activists, staged a peaceful sit-in at the office of Health Commissioner Stephen Joseph to protest what MHA member David Harris called "Joseph's malign neglect of widespread explicit educational efforts to stem the course of AIDS in favor of punitive measures scapegoating the most vulnerable and disenfranchised members of society." Their list of demands included "an end to Dr. Joseph's flailing about on the AIDS issue. Long-term planning is needed today to prepare for an excess of 100,000 New Yorkers who will have AIDS and AIDS-related illnesses by 1991. There is no time for false posturing on testing in an attempt to appear tough on the problem, while doing far too little to create workable solutions." Eight MHA members were arrested after Joseph refused to state publicly that he would reconsider his position.

What is really being tested? The limits of control that can be exerted over our bodies. The limits of constraint that can be placed on our actions.

We are being tested. The Reagan administration spends funds for costly, inefficient testing programs instead of for medical research, preventive education, and health care. This misuse of our tax dollars and neglect of our real needs tests the limits of our tolerance. It tests the limits of our will to fight back.

We in the communities affected by this epidemic will not stand for further intrusion into our already disempowered lives. Through direct action we will wrest control of the public discussion of AIDS. Through direct action we will make known the demands of the sick. Through direct action we will establish a national health care policy in the interests of people living with AIDS.

Drastic measures are being adopted. Activists are taking to the streets, making demands on their elected officials. Activists are providing alternative health care, educating their communities, researching alternative treatments. Activists are producing alternative media.

When circumstances require that drastic measures be adopted, independent media activists assume a central role. This role is twofold: to assist other activists in clarifying their positions and goals, and to represent those positions and goals to the world. Adopting the agenda of AIDS activists, media activists make armed propaganda.[2]

2. "The guerrilla expresses him or herself basically through armed activities, even if sometimes he or she uses other means of communication with people, like papers, pamphlets, radio messages, interference on radio and TV stations. . . . Armed propaganda takes on special importance . . . when it is a question of clarifying for the people, in periods when drastic measures must be adopted, positions whose goals are not sufficiently clear and which, thus, are difficult for the working-class mind to understand." Actas Tupamaras, "Tactics of the Urban Guerrilla" (1971), quoted in Armand Mattelart, "For a Class and Group Analysis of Popular Communication Practices," in

Video activists are everywhere met with the same challenges. We must call into question the established structures of the media. We must create new ways to make and distribute media. We must work toward participatory forms of representation that incorporate people into the communication process.

In the AIDS crisis, all of this must be done in order to facilitate moves toward the treatment and cure of AIDS, the distribution of preventive education materials, and the protection of civil rights. Video activists must clarify situations, render relations, picture possibilities for the emerging AIDS movement.

In the spring of 1987 the Testing the Limits collective, comprising lesbians, gays, and straights, formed to document emerging forms of activism developed in response to government inaction about the global AIDS epidemic. The founding members of the collective, Sandra Elgear, Robyn Hutt, Hilery Joy Kipnis, David Meieran, and myself, are all activists who view our documentary work as organizing work. The productive capacity and efficacy of the collective's project depends on establishing and

Seth Siegelaub and Armand Mattelart, eds., *Communication and Class Struggle, Liberation, Socialism*, vol. 2 (New York: International General, 1983), p. 20. Although the above quotation evidences voluntarist tendencies of revolutionary media theory regarding the "working-class mind," it adequately describes the radical potential of alternative media in times of struggle.

A war is being fought over our bodies. Thus, through civil disobedience we will use our bodies as means of contention. Continuing government inaction necessitates militancy. Even armed resistance may become necessary in response to widespread mandatory testing and/or quarantine.

maintaining links with protest-oriented groups and support organizations in the communities affected by AIDS.

Most of the members of the collective are participating members of ACT UP (AIDS Coalition to Unleash Power), "a diverse, nonpartisan group united in anger and committed to direct action to end the global AIDS epidemic." ACT UP's first action was staged on Wall Street in March 1987 to protest the unavailability of promising drug treatments and the announcement by Borroughs Wellcome that they would charge each patient up to $13,000 per year for AZT. Immediately following the action, at which seventeen people were arrested, the Food and Drug Administration announced plans to cut two years off the drug approval process. Media attention began to focus on drug treatment issues, and film of ACT UP's Wall Street demonstration became stock footage in subsequent reporting.

After this initial demonstration, ACT UP grew to be a core group of over 200 people. It coordinated the following actions in 1987:

[April 15: A demonstration at the Main Post Office in New York City protesting the lack of tax dollars earmarked for AIDS research.

[June 1: ACT UP joined other national activist organizations in civil disobedience at the White House. Washington police wore yellow rubber gloves as they arrested sixty-four people. Later that day, ACT UP demonstrated at the Third International Conference on AIDS. The civil disobedience garnered extensive international media attention. The second demonstration forced many public officials to break their seven-year silence.

[June 30: A rally and civil disobedience in Federal Plaza, New York City, to protest mandatory testing, immigration policy, and the negligence of the federal, state, and local governments. Thirty-three people were arrested.

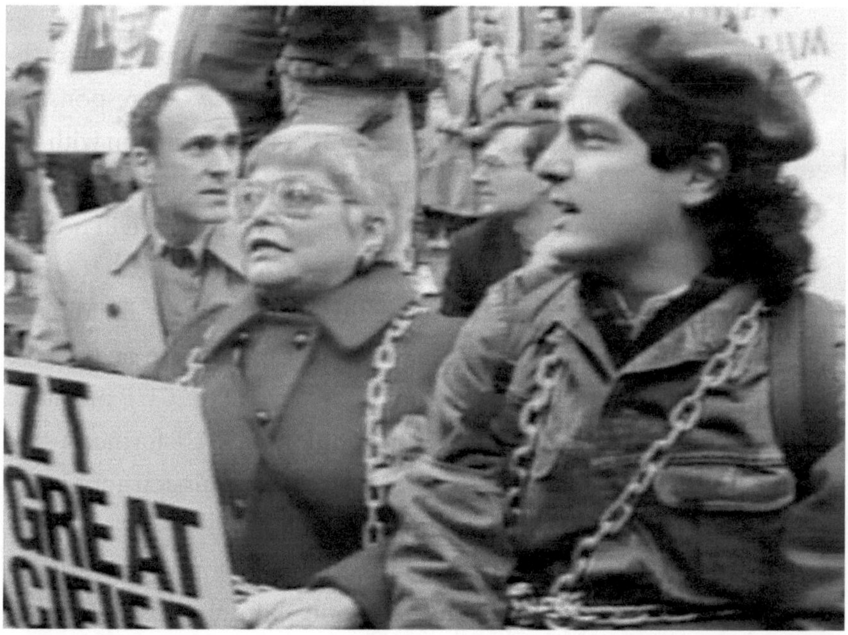

Figure 2.2 *Testing the Limits: New York,* Testing the Limits collective, 1987.

[July 21: A four-day, around-the-clock protest at Memorial Sloan-Kettering Hospital, one of the four AIDS Treatment Evaluation Units (ATEUs) in New York funded by the National Institutes of Health (NIH). ACT UP called for the NIH to conduct more clinical trials on promising drugs other than AZT and to increase the number of PLWAs in these trials. As a result of this demonstration, ACT UP established an ongoing dialogue with all four ATEUs in New York City.

[August 4: ACT UP quickly mobilized 100 people to protest Northwest Orient Airlines for refusing passage to PLWAs. In response to the demonstration and to lawsuits brought in conjunction with the Lambda Legal Defense League and the National Gay Rights Advocates, Northwest issued a policy statement that PLWAs will now be permitted to fly on the airline.

[September 9: A demonstration at the National Press Building in Washington, D.C., where the Presidential Commission on the HIV Epidemic was meeting for the first time. Several ACT UP members testified before the commission. In addition, ACT UP formed a subcommittee that continues to supply certain commission appointees with accurate and thorough information.

[September 22: ACT UP sponsored a community forum consisting of a twenty-member roundtable discussion about the possibilities for coordinated actions focused on issues of education, civil liberties, and health care.[3]

Through participation in ACT UP at every level of its process, the Testing the Limits collective has been able to document each of these

3. All information taken from an ACT UP pamphlet.

events, resulting in material that was, in effect, produced by the entire membership of ACT UP. As a member of both the video collective and the activist organization, it was important to me to be able to integrate my participation into a single practice. Thus, within ACT UP, I insisted that my work as a documentarian be recognized as itself a form of activism. Such recognition is hard-won. Activist groups generally consider only the dominant media, to which they have a fundamentally contradictory relationship: seeing it as the enemy and at the same time seeking legitimation from it. Discussions of the media are often bogged down in such petty issues as how to write a good press release or how to get the organization two minutes coverage on local news broadcasts.[4] An activist group that expends too much of its energy on the presentation of its image before the dominant media only gives the impression that it is more interested in publicity than in achieving its goals through direct action.

Within ACT UP, Testing the Limits had to earn its support. We were initially regarded as hobbyists, just as we are by the mainstream media: we cannot get press passes and the network musclemen physically cast us aside because we don't have broadcast-level equipment. One of our tasks therefore was to educate the group about the importance of alternative media. We had to introduce and reintroduce ourselves as independent documentarians within the group. We arranged screenings to show people what we were doing. We had constantly to announce our intentions and explain our activities.

Through this process, it became clear that the production of documentary overlaps with the efforts of political organizing. In order to tear down the structures that house the "public discussion" of AIDS, we have

4. See Dee Dee Halleck, "A Few Arguments for the Appropriation of Television," *High Performance* 37 (1987): 38–44.

to build alternative structures, structures that can generate and foster an affirmative culture for people living with AIDS.

As a member of ACT UP's Outreach Committee, I worked with others to establish relations with other AIDS activist and support groups. Such networking had also become the focus of Testing the Limits's project while documenting a teach-in, hosted by the *Village Voice,* at which many community representatives and groups were present. The collective also independently interviewed these organizations' members, including Suki Ports of the Minority Task Force on AIDS, Mitchell Karp of the Human Rights Commission's AIDS Discrimination Unit, and Yolanda Serrano of ADAPT (Association for Drug Abuse Prevention and Treatment).

The collective's videotaping coincided with and contributed to the work of the Outreach Committee in seeking to build a coalition between groups. In co-organizing the ACT UP-sponsored community forum in September 1987, I was able to get the participation of many of the community representatives with whom the collective had already worked. The community forum then generated still more documentary material, which was edited by Jean Carlomusto, producer of Gay Men's Health Crisis's cable program *Living with AIDS,* into a half-hour show broadcast on the program the following week.

All the material the collective produced within the first three months after its formation was compiled into a six-minute tape. Entitled *Testing the Limits,* the tape is a fast-paced trailer that serves as a short catalog of resistance to government policy.[5] It draws on the experiences of people from many communities affected by the AIDS crisis. Taped in various so-

5. The pilot was first described as a "catalog of resistance" by Mark Dion. The designation is appropriate because the pilot tape is an "index" to the kinds of direct action being taken as well as to the documentary material that constitutes the tape.

cial spaces around New York, people are shown in meeting halls, churches, parks, homes, in the studio, at rallies, demonstrations, forums.

Testing the Limits is scripted to the song "Living in Wartime" written by Michael Callen, a person living with AIDS and founding member of the PWA Coalition, and performed by the group Low Life.

> This is the time for doubting,
> To stop and wonder why.
> This is the time for shouting
> I don't believe the lies.
> One way or another
> No one will be spared.
> Call out to my brothers
> Doesn't anybody care?
> We are living,
> We are living in wartime.[6]

This song was used as a vehicle to organize information and propel the viewer through the material. "Living in Wartime" figures far more significantly in the tape than merely as a sound track. Both lyrics and melody are used as a formal, rhetorical structure that narrativizes the roughly compiled material within the tape. The song functions to organize the dense arrangement of information, shaping it into a work of propaganda. This tape is an attempt to use the music television form—a commodity form—as a form of truly popular culture. We appropriated some of the tropes of MTV to deploy them as agit-prop.

6. "Living in Wartime," music and lyrics by Michael Callen, performed by Low Life, © Tops and Bottoms, Inc., BMI.

The six-minute tape was used effectively as an organizing tool, screened in galleries, at meetings, fundraisers, and on cable TV. It was also screened at the lesbian and gay film festivals in San Francisco, Chicago, and New York. In addition, it functioned as a pilot for the collective's future documentary projects.

Testing the Limits, the pilot tape, would become a model for a twenty-eight minute video called *Testing the Limits: New York.* Like the pilot, this tape is a catalog of resistance drawn from the nearly 100 hours of video the collective had produced. The collective made the decision to edit the material according to voice, as opposed to image. We wanted to listen to what people had to say about themselves and their situations.

Statements by activists from many communities were roughly ordered according to three areas of concern in the AIDS crisis: civil liberties, education, and health care. The script was divided into three sections according to these categories, recognizing that each of the categories would be triangulated around every issue, within each section. The collective discussed the many varied points of view expressed in the material and arrived at editing decisions through a loose consensus process. We arranged and rearranged clusters of material according to the particular relation of each of the members to the issues. Our task was complicated, sometimes painful, as our decisions had to be mediated by the multiplicity of social relations in play.

This collective process resulted in a number of awkward juxtapositions within the tape. One of the most jarring occurred in the section on education, in which a statement by Ruth Rodriguez of the Hispanic AIDS Forum was followed by a statement by Denise Ribble of the Community Health Project. Speaking in Spanish (subtitled in English), Rodriguez delivers an impassioned speech to members of her own community on issues of Latino representation and self-determination. Immediately following, Ribble describes the use of dental dams in lesbian safe-sex practices. The conflict of the two segments involves more than the obvious. Rodriguez directly addresses the camera with a sense of rage. Then, relaxed in her clinical setting and clearly talking about something she enjoys, Ribble presents to the camera a piece of green latex, her "Christmas version" of the dental dam.

It is difficult to articulate what disturbed us about this juxtaposition. To my mind, we were confronted by our own internalized homophobia. We didn't think that a description of lesbian sexual practices should follow a statement about the cultural exclusion of the Latino community. We were afraid to risk offending the Latino community, assuming that that community would not view the issues as of equivalent importance.

This discomfort evidenced a historically specific discursive formation. For the sake of countering prevalent assumptions, such as "AIDS is a gay disease," many activists will deny that their sexual orientation is associated with their AIDS activism. This is counterbalanced by others who stress the problems the epidemic has posed for certain gay people to such an extent that they exclude recognition of the problems for anyone else. Regardless of intention, I think the collective, at times, recapitulated the homophobia exemplified by the former tendency. I think we experienced our own internalized AIDS-related homophobia. But there's no such thing as a thought crime. Editing occasioned a process that enabled us to work through some of the specular relations implicit in AIDS work. For me, each image that raised issues of sexuality was charged with questions about my own sexual orientation. I was forced to consider issues of race, gender, and class as they figure in relation to gay sexual politics.

The juxtaposition of Ruth Rodriguez's statement and Denise Ribble's description did not seem to make sense at all, even though we had arrived at it through a reasoned process. In fact, what *does* make sense in the AIDS crisis would, in other circumstances, seem a non sequitur. The current situation involves a collision of issues that had existed before the epidemic. The response to the epidemic has thus enabled a number of groups to understand social injustices as systemic biases within society that affect all subaltern groups differently. For this reason, the experience of various issues by diverse groups must be rendered in terms of the common situation. Further, this compilation of experiences must be shown to result in a sense of shared goals.

In the end, we didn't retain the Rodriguez–Ribble juxtaposition. Other combinations of material seemed to approximate the historical conditions more accurately, according to the consensus of the collective. The entire section on education became a collage in which issues of cultural sensitivity are formally anchored by Denise Ribble's safe sex instructions. These instructions are edited to intervene at regular intervals that determine the pace of what would otherwise seem arbitrary in the arrangement of material in the section. We arrived at this formal solution in view of our historical situation: experiences were grounded in a presentation of the principles of safe sex practices.

Editing decisions show the rough composition of issues that are the AIDS crisis, triangulated around civil liberties, education, and health care. This multiplicity is rendered—as voiced—by members of the affected communities. Concerns specific to each community are roughly juxtaposed. The single most important objective is to affirm the lives of people living with AIDS and the social relations these lives include. Finally, it is necessary to show courses of action that will bring about positive change. Protest and resistance must be militantly advocated.

Testing the Limits: New York is punctuated with powerful images of protest, explicitly intended to present direct action as the means to change. References to the print media and network television are occasionally introduced to situate the issues polemically in relation to the so-called public discussion of AIDS. The use of music serves a similar purpose, attempting to ground the tape in genuinely popular cultural production.

"Living in Wartime," the song used for the pilot, opened and closed the twenty-eight minute tape.

> They try to break our spirits.
> They try to keep us in our place.
> They do it to the women
> And the poor of every race.
> We face a common enemy,
> Bigotry and greed.
> But if we fight together
> We will find the strength we need.
> We are living,
> We are living in wartime.[7]

A section of the rap called "Respect Yourself," produced by the Philadelphia AIDS Task Force, was used in a transition between the section on civil liberties and that on education. The transition is a quick-paced, diced selection of urban images contrasted with images of protest. Scripted

7. Ibid.

with a simple theme of "movement" in mind, it is roughly edited to the rap beat.

> Be you a butcher, a baker, a candlestick maker,
> AIDS don't care about the color of your skin.
> You gotta keep your body strong.
> Respect yourself and you will live long.[8]

The only other scored transition occurs between the sections on education and health care. A portion of the Romanovsky and Philips song "Homophobia" is played under a series of images about "touch." Shots of the Washington police wearing rubber gloves at a protest are paired with images of activists joining hands at the ACT UP civil disobedience at Federal Plaza in New York.

> Now AIDS has claimed so many lives
> And still there is no cure,
> And if they don't spend more on research
> It will keep on killing more.
> Because it's called a gay disease
> It's easy to ignore,
> Which sounds a lot like blatant homophobia to me.[9]

Songs can succinctly render complex concerns in ways that are extremely accessible; music-making is central to building a popular culture.

8. "Respect Yourself," produced by Philadelphia Community Health Alternatives, Black and White Men Together, with the assistance of the US Conference of Mayors.
9. "Homophobia," music and lyrics by Romanovsky and Philips, © 1985 Romanovsky and Philips. Thanks for their continuing commitment to lesbian and gay activism.

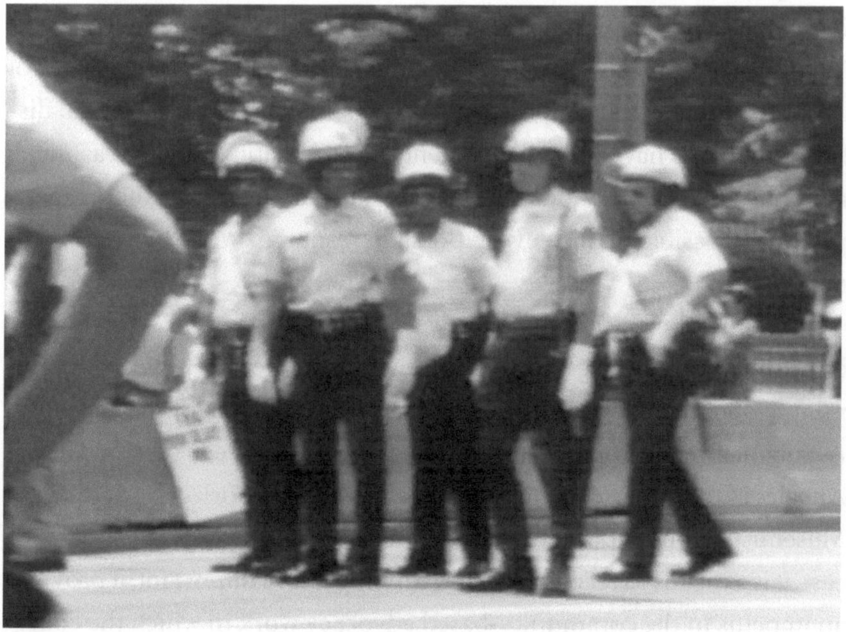

Figure 2.3 *Testing the Limits: New York,* Testing the Limits collective, 1987.

As we scripted sections of the tape to this music, it became clear that the collective's activity is part of an emerging cultural project.

The agenda of this project compels the video activist to organize the screening and distribution of material. People must be able to see themselves making history. People living with AIDS must be able to see themselves not as victims, but as self-empowered activists. In view of this agenda, distribution plans have to be fundamentally pragmatic: Generate as much material as possible. Show this material in as many forms and as many places as possible. Utilize every possible resource. Work by any means necessary.

The Testing the Limits collective has addressed issues of distribution by organizing its production as a self-generating process. The twenty-eight-minute documentary is the "public image" for the work of the collective. As such, it is made to appeal to a wide audience. It has been screened in Los Angeles at the American Film Institute and in New York at both the New Museum of Contemporary Art and Global Village. Appropriate for broadcast, it is a means to recognition and funding. More important, it provides an impetus to the community-based advocacy work in which the collective is engaged. Our material can be disseminated through local distribution, presented anywhere a screening is possible. The collective has a policy of sharing material with anyone in the movement. Aside from the local VCR circuit, material is fed to public access programs such as *Living with AIDS*, mentioned above, and *Out in the Eighties*, a gay cable TV show. It is possible to set up screenings anywhere. Some groups have organized screenings in parking lots, running tapes off the cigarette lighter of a station wagon, propping the TV on the tailgate.[10]

Imagine a screening. In a local community center a consumer VCR deck and a TV set sit on a table. Representatives from the various communities affected by AIDS sit in front of the TV. They watch a video composed of interviews with each of them. They see themselves pictured in relation to one another as they sit next to one another.

Consider this screening. It presents both means and ends for the video AIDS activist. The AIDS movement, like other radical movements, creates itself as it attempts to represent itself. Video puts into play the means of recognizing one's place within the movement in relation to that of others in the movement. Video has the potential to render the concerted efforts—as yet unimagined—between groups. The most significant challenge to the movement is coalition building, because the AIDS epidemic has engendered a community of people who cannot afford *not* to recognize themselves as a community and to act as one.

The AIDS epidemic has caused us to change our behavior. It has shaped our social relations as it has changed our views of ourselves. This became apparent to me recently, after coming out to my family. I realized that I had come out as a member of two disenfranchised groups. I am a member of the gay community and a member of the AIDS community. Furthermore, I am a gay member of the AIDS community, a community that some would establish by force, for no other end but containment, toward no other end but repression, with no other end but our deaths—a community that must, instead, establish *itself* in the face of this containment and repression. We must proudly identify ourselves as a coalition.

10. See Halleck, "A Few Arguments," p. 40.

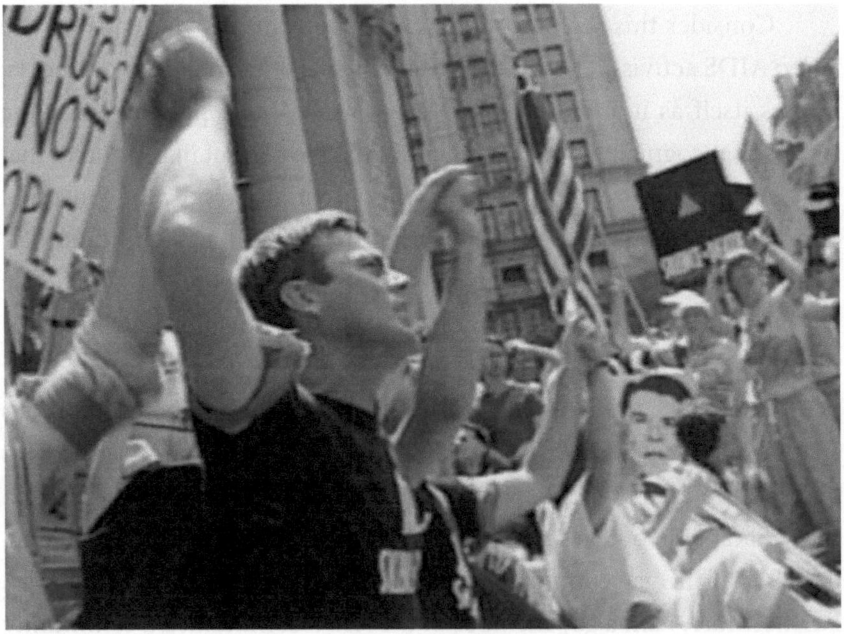

Figure 2.4 *Testing the Limits: New York,* Testing the Limits collective, 1987.

Picture a coalition of people refusing to be victims.

Picture a coalition of people distributing condoms and clean works.

Picture a coalition of people having safe sex and shooting up with clean works.

Picture a coalition of people staging a die-in in front of City Hall or the White House until massive funds for AIDS are released.

Picture a coalition of people getting arrested for blocking traffic during rush hour as they stand in the middle of Times Square kissing one another.

Picture a coalition of people occupying abandoned buildings, demanding that they be made into hospices for people living with AIDS.

Picture a coalition of people chanting "Money for AIDS, not for war" as they surround and quarantine the Pentagon.

The government and the medical establishment denounce as "immoral" the people who get sick and the people they hope will get sick. They worry about themselves, their children, and the "innocent victims." They predict the kinds of people who get AIDS, the numbers of people infected, the numbers of deaths that will occur. But they are doing next to nothing to cure the sick and prevent the spread of AIDS.

People are asking, "If they won't do anything now, when will they?" "If they won't do anything for those who are sick now, for whom will they?"

Getting no answers, people are mobilizing.

Getting no answers, a movement is emerging.

Picture a coalition of people who *will* end this epidemic.

The AIDS Crisis Is Ridiculous

3

In memory of Craig Owens

Originally published as "The AIDS Crisis Is Ridiculous," *Queer Looks*, eds. Martha Gever, John Greyson, and Prahtiba Parmar (London, New York: Routledge, 1993), pp. 208–224. Minor revisions have been made for consistency. Reproduced by permission of Routledge/Taylor & Francis Books, Inc.

MANIFESTO

Ridiculous Theater,
Scourge of Human Folly
by
Charles Ludlam

Aim: To get beyond nihilism by revaluing combat.

Axioms to a theater for ridicule:

1. You are a living mockery of your own ideals. If not, you have set your ideals too low.
2. The things one takes seriously are one's weaknesses.
3. Just as many people who claim a belief in God disprove it with their every act, so too there are those whose every deed, though they say there is no God, is an act of faith.
4. Evolution is a conscious process.
5. Bathos is that which is intended to be sorrowful but because of the extremity of its expression becomes comic. Pathos is that which is meant to be comic but because of the extremity of its expression becomes sorrowful. Some things which seem to be opposites are actually different degrees of the same thing.
6. The comic hero thrives by his vices. The tragic hero is destroyed by his virtue. Moral paradox is the crux of the drama.
7. The theater is a humble materialist enterprise which seeks to produce riches of the imagination, not the other way around. The theater is an event and not an object. Theater workers need not blush and conceal their desperate struggle to pay the landlords their rents. Theater without the stink of art.

"*Instructions for use:*
This is farce not Sunday school. Illustrate hedonistic calculus. Test out a dangerous idea, a theme that threatens to destroy one's whole value system. Treat the material in a madly farcical manner without losing the seriousness of the theme. Show how paradoxes arrest the mind. Scare yourself a bit along the way."

The only thing that is different from one time to another is what is seen and what is seen depends upon how everybody is doing everything. This makes the thing we are looking at very different and this makes what those who describe it make of it, it makes a composition, it confuses, it shows, it is, it looks, it likes it as it is, and this makes what is seen as it is seen. Nothing changes from generation to generation except the thing seen and that makes a composition. —*Gertrude Stein*[1]

Chapter 3 *The AIDS Crisis Is Ridiculous*

[A Fantasy about a Father]

Charles Ludlam died of pneumonia on Friday, May 29, 1987, at St. Vincent's Hospital in New York City at about 1 A.M. just after his longtime lover Everett Quinton had left his bedside. He had recently been diagnosed with AIDS, and his death stunned our community, which is still

1. Gertrude Stein, "Composition as Explanation," in Carl Van Vechten, ed., *Selected Writings* (New York: Random House, 1962), p. 516.

struggling daily with the devastation of AIDS. My relation to Ludlam and his theater is particular to the historical circumstances of the AIDS crisis. I never met him, and I never saw him perform. When he died, I became part of a local, collective remembrance of this almost mythic gay figure. I recently attended the opening night of the Ridiculous Theater Company's newest production of *Camille,* on my birthday. Everett Quinton performed in the role that Ludlam made famous. I could not resist viewing the final scene as about Ludlam's death and Quinton's mourning.

> [H]e was not, as has wrongly been assumed by the daily press, an avant-garde artist in the least; he was the reviver and purifier of a thousand traditions that had fallen into corruption, banality, and disrepute. He reinvented the burlesque tradition, the vaudeville and silent-film tradition of physical comedy, the tradition of playwrighting as an ongoing conversation with a faithful audience, the tradition of repertory acting.[2]

I know some details of Ludlam's life and career only through reading obituaries, yet I have a fantasy: I am having dinner with Charles Ludlam in a West Village restaurant, telling him about an article I am writing about AIDS-activist video. He seems intrigued, but actually he is humoring me. He thinks I'm a cute kid, and he's interested in getting into my pants. I'd let him. This is a fantasy about lineage. I desire a link with Ludlam, a link with the past, a place in history. There must be some continuity between our lives, and if not our lives, the history and the forces that have shaped them.

> When Ludlam turned, in *Camille,* to his maid in a boudoir in Paris and said (in that ruminating pathetic tone), "Throw another faggot

2. Michael Feingold, "The Great Continuum," *Village Voice,* June 9, 1987, p. 88.

> on the fire!" whole ages of repression went up in shrieks. "There are no faggots in the house Madame," the maid replied respectfully. And Ludlam—rising on one arm on the chaise lounge to look directly out at the audience with that affable expression—would say, "What? No faggots in the house?"
>
> There were lots of faggots in the house, of course—bronzed, muscular habitues of gyms, muscles, and mustaches—and if everything Ludlam did was ironic, a double entendre of sorts, so were their lives.[3]

In my fantasy I want Ludlam to fuck me without a condom. I'd receive his cure as a gift. Searching for a model, I wish for a legacy—the love and approval of a father. I want to achieve his stature. In my fantasy, Ludlam's greatness can be passed on to me through his semen. A condom would thwart this transference. This is a fantasy about immortality; that something exists greater than ourselves, shared between us—our community, for example.

> Excess was Charles Ludlam's point of departure, his first gift. He knew that what was attainable in reality was always within theater's reach. Castration, gender flops, defloration, psychotic episodes, and curtain-chewing were not only possible but commonplace at the Ridiculous Theater. Harder than imagining Ludlam—outsized, operatic, a force of theater and life—in a truly tragic role is knowing that we will never again see him waggle a dildo across the footlights or cock an eyebrow and stage lisp "I love my makeup tonight."[4]

3. Andrew Holleran, "New York Notebook: Tragic Drag," *Christopher Street* 113 (July, 1987): 12.
4. Guy Trebay, "The Gift of Excess," *Village Voice,* June 9, 1987, p. 98.

My fantasy raises a number of issues regarding AIDS and HIV transmission. I am well aware of the implications of this fantasy. I am HIV antibody positive, and I was infected through unprotected sexual intercourse. Today I use condoms to protect myself from any number of infections that can threaten my already-compromised immune system. Yet I still dream about unsafe sex. When I tested HIV antibody positive in the spring of 1988, at twenty-four years old, I no longer felt part of my generation of gay men. I felt like a member of a past generation. My fantasy reveals that, unconsciously, I think that AIDS is the legacy I have inherited from the previous generation of gay men. It is difficult not to blame past lovers for my HIV infection, regardless of the fact that I know that no one is to blame—my lovers or myself. It has been equally difficult not to understand my HIV infection as a punishment, regardless of my sex radicalism. The hardest thing I have had to accept is that there is no reason that explains AIDS. There are historical, material conditions that create a situation of crisis, but there is no reason why some people die, why some get sick, why I am infected. There is no reason, but there is meaning. My experiences are filled with meaning. They're filled with pain, irony, and hope.[5]

Thus, I am motivated to establish a comparative relation between Ludlam's theater project and the growing body of video work to which I have contributed. This relation is somewhat implausible. Ludlam intended to make people laugh, but the intention of AIDS-activist video is to make people angry. The Ridiculous Theater is studiedly apolitical, while most AIDS-activist video work is propagandistic. Yet, I can conceive of a relation with Ludlam within what can be described as a psycho-geographic proximity. We exist in the same place at different times. Remember Gertrude Stein's words, "Nothing changes from generation to generation

5. I would like to thank Peter Bowen, Jeff Nunokawa, Michael Perelman, and Daniel Wolfe for discussing this fantasy with me and for helping me to understand it.

except the thing seen and that makes a composition." Consider that "the thing seen" is the AIDS epidemic.

[Queer Structures of Feeling]

There are countercultural strategies that belong specifically to queers. A queer structure of feeling shapes cultural work produced by queers. In the words of Raymond Williams, who coined the term, a structure of feeling is "the hypothesis of a mode of social formation, explicit and recognizable in specific kinds of art, which is distinguishable from other social and semantic formations by its articulations of presence."[6]

Within the relation between two factors, a queer structure of feeling is formed. These two factors are: how heterosexist oppression attempts to contain queer sexualities, and how queers fight oppression by forming communities. Thus, a queer structure of feeling can be described as an articulation of presence forged through resistance to heterosexist society. Cultural work can be considered within a queer structure of feeling if self-identified queers produce the work, if these producers identify the work as queer, if queers claim the work has significance to queers, if the work is censored or criticized for being queer. A particular work is queer if it is viewed as queer, either by queers or bigots.

A queer structure of feeling is a set of cultural strategies of survival for queers. It is marked by an appreciation for the ridiculous, and it values masquerade. Mockery is its form; posing is its strategy. These general terms describe a continuity in the structure that traverses a number of generations. From generation to generation the emphasis of the structure

6. Raymond Williams, *Marxism and Literature* (Oxford and New York: Oxford University Press, 1977), p. 135.

shifts and new articulations surface to define the current moment. Some of the defining characteristics remain present in new articulations, establishing continuities in form.

The AIDS epidemic precipitated a crisis affecting the actual conditions of existence of many artists—many of them gay. Thus, many lesbian and gay artists took ideas current in the art world—appropriation, situationist strategies, institutional critique—and applied them to the struggle to wrest control of the public discussion of AIDS from right-wing fanatics who proposed homophobic and racist policies like quarantine. AIDS media activists also steal methods from dominant culture to make work that is meaningful to the communities affected by AIDS. Additionally, these activists deploy strategies that have been used effectively by lesbians and gay men to fight invisibility. These strategies are what Ridiculous Theater and AIDS-activist video share in common.

[Material Conditions]

Ludlam considers the material conditions of production:

> The theater is a humble materialist enterprise which seeks to produce riches of the imagination, not the other way around. The theater is an event not an object. Theater workers need not blush and conceal their desperate struggle to pay the landlords their rents. Theater without the stink of art.

Without access to substantial resources, AIDS video activists have organized around principles similar to those underlying Ludlam's seventh axiom. It is recognized that video "is not an object, but an event," because its production is part of a larger effort to organize increasing numbers of people to take action. Video "without the stink of art" is television. We are not primarily concerned with video as a form. The production of activist video is primarily concerned with audience and distribution. Many people who make video do not have access to airtime or broadcast-quality equipment. Despite the lack of access to substantial resources, AIDS activists make television which is radically different from that of the network television industry, where the only motivation is profit.

Among many AIDS video activists, video production is viewed as a collaborative effort, recognizing that material conditions dictate the form of production. Video production is a means to end government inaction on AIDS. This agenda compels activists to put work in as many places and in as many forms as possible. AIDS activist video is produced in a dialogue with the social movement to end government inaction. The documentation of protests is one form of direct action; distributions of these tapes are demonstrations.

[Video Ridiculous]

There are elements of the aesthetics of Ridiculous Theater to be found in current AIDS-activist video production, but there are no direct correlations. Current queer video practices draw on the history of queer theater of the seventies, adding to it the political agendas of AIDS activism and lesbian and gay liberation as they are presently articulated and understood. In this way a new queer structure of feeling is articulated. The following considers aspects of the ridiculous that can be located in some AIDS activist videos. Each of the videos discussed here exemplifies different aspects of the current queer structure of feeling.

Stiff Sheets (1989), by John Goss, presents a video record of a theatrical performance by AIDS activists. From January 21 to 28, 1989, ACT UP Los Angeles staged a continual vigil at L.A. County/University of Southern California Medical Center to protest the government's lethally slow response to AIDS. The protestors demanded the immediate creation of AIDS services and facilities. On the sixth evening of the vigil, an anonymous collective of gay artists, using the pseudonym Stiff Sheets, presented a fashion show to entertain the demonstrators.

The master of ceremonies started the show with "a little polite disclaimer," stating, "This fashion show is brought to you in the worst taste imaginable, and you are the most sensitized of audiences imaginable. So, if you are offended we are too." This is significant for two reasons. First, it aligns the performance within the history of queer theater—particularly Ridiculous Theater—by acknowledging its intentions to mine the depths of bad taste. Additionally, it acknowledges a specific audience of AIDS activists who will appreciate the humor in a particular way.

The performance acknowledged both the rage of the activists and some of the most morbid aspects of living with AIDS. For example, in a scene featuring "active sportswear," a model walks down the runway wearing a sweatshirt and sweatpants. The MC announces that the creation is titled "night sweats—more than a fashion, it's a condition; more than a style, it's a symptom." Another outfit presented was an ankle-length pink triangle with the slogan "SILENCE = DEATH" printed along the bottom. "When the epidemic started getting out of hand and no other gay organization responded to the great fashion needs required, we made the transition from checkbook activism and took to the streets," comments the MC. The irony here depends on stereotypical views of gay men as stylish, or as drag queens, coupled with an awareness that a pink triangle accompanied by the SILENCE = DEATH logo *is* a fashion statement about the

AIDS epidemic. The outfit, then, underscores the strategic role of style for AIDS activists.

A third ensemble modeled in the tape reveals changes in queer structures of feeling concerned with gay male sexuality. During the "bridal finale" two contrasting examples are presented. Last decade's look appears as a model dressed in a tattered bridal gown decorated with clumps of hardened sperm. Carrying wilted flowers, the old queen drags her tired ass down the aisle to make way for the chic and fabulous safe-sex bride of the eighties. Dressed in a white gown tightly bound with Saran wrap, this eager girl wears leather underwear, and she is prepared to have safe sex, "enabling her to stay alive for the divorce."

DiAna's Hair Ego, AIDS Info Up Front (1990), by Ellen Spiro, describes the efforts of the South Carolina AIDS Education Network (SCAEN)—a grassroots organization based in the salon, DiAna's Hair Ego. Here, the shop's owner, beautician DiAna DiAna, provides education about AIDS to all her clients. Printed matter and condoms are made available on shelves displaying beauty products; educational tapes are screened on a television monitor in the salon. The situation depicted in *DiAna's Hair Ego* is implicitly theatrical, a quality further emphasized by Spiro's documentation. Various shots of the beauty shop are recorded with a wide-angle lens, giving it the appearance of a fishbowl and suggesting that this site of community activism can be viewed microcosmically as a model for what AIDS education should be—a grassroots effort designed by a community in its own interests. Spiro's camera direction is very theatrical at times. She wasn't intimidated by the mirrors in the beauty shop and didn't shy away from images that show her reflection in the shop's mirrors.

Spiro's incorporation of the activity of documentation in the tape echoes SCAEN's use of performance for AIDS education. DiAna is shown making presentations about AIDS at local conferences and directing others in role-playing exercises designed to address the complex issues of negotiating safer sex. Spiro also includes footage shot by DiAna of local schoolchildren asking questions about AIDS: "Can you get it from mosquitos?" "Why isn't a cure found?" "Do more blacks get AIDS than whites?" Employing a multitude of devices that complement SCAEN's efforts, *DiAna's Hair Ego* demonstrates the nexus of theater, video, and AIDS activism.

Bob Huff's *Rockville Is Burning* (1989), perhaps the most successful hybrid of Ridiculous Theater and video activism to date, is based on a performance about an AIDS-activist takeover of a network television news program. The performance included the use of video within the structure of the play, and both the performance and the videotaped material are set against the background of the ACT UP/ACT NOW nonviolent takeover of the Food and Drug Administration (FDA) headquarters in Rockville, Maryland on October 11, 1988. This theater piece was the product of collaboration between Bob Huff and an ACT UP affinity group, Wave Three. Theater became one of their activities when they were invited to present a work at La Mama, ETC in Manhattan.

In the opening scene, an effeminate, implied closet-case director coaches a newscaster about the tone he should affect when presenting the news that AIDS activists have occupied the FDA building. He convinces the newscaster to agree to be more sympathetic to the protesters, explaining that the enormous, and increasing, number of people with AIDS and HIV "represents significant demographics." However, on the air the news-

caster adopts a sensational tone and refers to the AIDS activists as "a group of homosexual protestors," a cliché common in the broadcast industry that has contributed to the misperception that AIDS is a "gay disease."

In the middle of the newscaster's presentation of the FDA action, three "AIDS terrorists" in white lab coats burst onto the set, announcing that they have taken control. Supposedly, other "AIDS terrorists" have control of the network's satellite transponder, enabling them to interrupt the news to receive transmissions from around the country. These segments consist of interviews Huff had previously recorded, with members of Wave Three playing different "AIDS victims"—an IV drug user, a mother, a person with AIDS, a hemophiliac, a child—each enacted as a drag performance.

This dramatized reworking of mass media representations in *Rockville Is Burning,* seen from an activist's perspective, fulfills many fantasies. Videotaping himself in his newscaster persona, superimposed on images of the actual action at the FDA, Huff reports a riot. Archival images of people rioting and buildings burning are likewise presented as live footage from the FDA action. This projection of riots, armed takeovers, and even assassinations represents the frustration of AIDS activists faced with the slow response of government institutions to the epidemic. It also represents the ongoing debates about the options open to the AIDS-activist movement; until now AIDS activists have relied on nonviolent direct action to achieve their ends. Huff's tape pushes the boundaries of the continuing discussion concerning tactics in ways reminiscent of Ridiculous Theater. As Ludlam advises, "Test out a dangerous idea, a theme which threatens to destroy one's whole value system," and "Treat the material in a madly farcical manner without losing the seriousness of the theme."

[Sorrow]

For Ludlam, sorrow is at the center of drama:

> Bathos is that which is intended to be sorrowful but because of the extremity of the expression becomes comic. Pathos is that which is meant to be comic but because of the extremity of its expression

becomes sorrowful. Some things which seem to be opposites are actually different degrees of the same thing.

But there is nothing intrinsically sorrowful about being queer. Oppression causes the sorrow in the lives of queers, and queers have developed a rich culture filled with joy in the face of sorrow. In particular, many AIDS media activists have organized into collectives, sharing resources to produce work vital to the interests of the communities affected by AIDS. I am a founding member of two AIDS video collectives: the Testing the Limits collective, formed in 1987 to document emerging forms of AIDS activism and which produced a videotape of the same name; and DIVA TV (Damned Interfering Video Activists), an affinity group of ACT UP that documents actions and provides countersurveillance against police brutality at demonstrations. This loosely organized collective of approximately thirty members has produced three tapes thus far—*Target City Hall, Pride,* and *Like a Prayer* (all 1989). Both collectives use democratic forms, such as consensus decision-making. The goals of both collectives are to quickly produce tapes that can be used by AIDS-activist direct action groups as organizing tools.

The processes employed by these collectives are significantly different from those found in the repertory theater. The Ridiculous Theatrical Company was a small ensemble, under Ludlam's direction, committed to changing the history of theater. During the AIDS crisis there is no sense that one can afford to work for years with a small group of people developing a set of ideas. And, although AIDS-activist collectives have their share of divas, they are leaderless. They function with an extreme sense of urgency. A number of collective members in DIVA have died from AIDS and many people, in both video groups, have lost numerous friends and lovers. Many AIDS activists are sick or HIV-infected. It is not possible for these groups to conceive of working relationships that aren't focused on well-defined, pragmatic goals that can be achieved in relatively short periods of time.

The production of *Target City Hall* addressed this imperative in its design as a work comprising sections, each produced by a different group with different levels of experience. The tape documented ACT UP's efforts to take over City Hall in New York in the late winter of 1989, in order to call attention to the collapse of the city's health care system. A music video section introduces the documentary. Another section, produced by the late Costa Pappas, draws on conventions of direct cinema and cinema verité. The third section was made by a group of lesbians who adopted the name LAPIT (Lesbian Activists Producing Innovative Television) and whose contribution uses images from commercial TV news broadcasts juxtaposed with interviews, performances, rap, and activist-produced protest footage. Interspersed between these segments, the collective's editing committee added scenes, shot on black-and-white Super 8 film, of AIDS activists getting arrested at City Hall, which resemble archival footage of civil rights protests or demonstrations against U.S. involvement in Vietnam. A full inventory of the conventions and tropes used in *Target City Hall* reflects the conflicting feelings of desperation and hopefulness that inform a queer structure of feeling, as well as a willingness to try any approach that will achieve a desired effect. This was true for Ludlam, and it is also true for many queer videomakers producing work about AIDS: "The theater absurd believes in nothing, the theater ridiculous believes in everything."[7]

The queer theft of straight culture must not be viewed merely as oppositional. Ridiculous Theater, too, "is not a comment (nostalgic, ironic,

7. Richard Elovich tells me that he saw this statement on a poster advertising a Ridiculous production in the seventies.

adoring, or patronizing) on mass culture but it borrows from and imitates mass culture as fellow product of the popular imagination."[8] It is possible to feel both admiration and contempt for dominant culture, and queers may easily have contradictory feelings about the culture that ignores and ridicules us. We are not acknowledged, nor are we invited to participate in this culture, but we comprise part of its audience. In his careful, studied use of material stolen from dominant culture—movies, plays, television, magazines, newspapers—Ludlam revealed a fascination with it. However, his use of this material was not destructive; it was generative. According to Ludlam, the aim of Ridiculous Theater is "to get beyond nihilism by revaluing combat." Today's videomakers manipulate the stuff that has fascinated us all our television-watching lives. For AIDS activists, getting "beyond nihilism" requires that we overcome cynicism about our role in historical change. By "revaluing combat" we assume responsibility toward change, recognizing our stake in dominant culture along the way.

Where Ludlam offers "instructions for use" of his manifesto, he counsels, "This is farce not Sunday school." This thought is useful when considering AIDS activists' efforts to criticize religious institutions as documented in the DIVA production *Like a Prayer.* The video chronicles the Stop the Church demonstration organized by ACT UP New York and WHAM! (Women's Health Action Movement) at St. Patrick's Cathedral on September 10, 1989, to protest the Catholic Church's—specifically Cardinal John O'Connor's—opposition to women's right to choose abortion and everybody's right to use condoms.

In this work, we find an overt overlap between Ludlam's theater practice and AIDS activism in Operation Ridiculous, a WHAM! affinity group whose name and actions parody Operation Rescue, the right-

8. Stefan Brecht, *Queer Theater* (London and New York: Methuen, 1978), p. 48.

wing antichoice group that blocks women's access to abortion clinics. The DIVA tape shows members of Operation Rescue holding pictures of fetuses and carrying rubber models of fetuses at different stages of development. In parallel sequences, the Operation Ridiculous group arrives at the demonstration in clown suits holding dolls dressed as "clown babies" and screeching, "Save the babies! Save our clown babies." The affinity group intervenes wherever members of Operation Rescue gather to disrupt the protest at St. Patrick's.

As these images appear on screen, members of Operation Ridiculous proclaim:

> It's ridiculous that Operation Rescue, a predominantly white group, preaches carrying all pregnancies to term while there are over thirty thousand babies waiting to be adopted, the majority of whom are babies of color.
>
> It's ridiculous that the Catholic Church actively blocks safe sex and birth control education in the schools. Teenagers are exceptionally active. They're getting pregnant, and there has been a forty-percent rise in teenage AIDS cases.
>
> It's ridiculous that dialogue on reproductive rights has been limited to abortion when real issues like the lack of prenatal, neonatal, and gynecological care are virtually ignored.
>
> It's ridiculous that the Catholic Church preaches brotherly love yet promotes antigay and antilesbian violence by calling homosexuality a sin.

In *Like a Prayer,* Operation Ridiculous exhibits a keen sense of the ridiculous, combined with a sophisticated understanding of direct action, bringing to mind Ludlam's axiom:

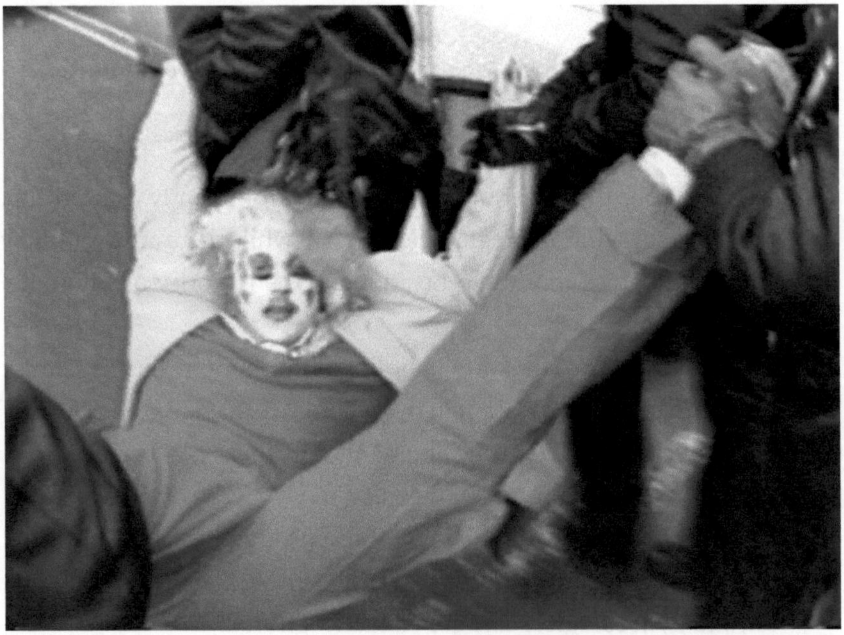

Figure 3.1 *Like a Prayer,* DIVA TV, 1989.

> Just as many people who claim a belief in God disprove it with their very act, so too there are those whose every deed, though they say there is no God, is an act of faith.

[Sex and Virtue]

Ludlam describes religious paradox as a means to question all moral order: "Illustrate hedonistic calculus." The performers of Ridiculous Theater have been described as "erotic beings intent on self-affirmation."[9] Several AIDS-activist videos begin with the same premise.

In *Keep Your Laws Off My Body* (1989), by Zoe Leonard and Catherine Saalfield, images of two lesbians having sex are juxtaposed with shots of uniformed police officers at an ACT UP demonstration. More romantic than ridiculous, the slow pans caressing the women's flesh reveal that this material was shot by the two women. Stiff, overdressed, stuffy, and nervous, the lines of uniformed cops stare in one direction; sometimes they look directly into the camera. The alternating presence and absence of the lesbian lovers and the legion of law enforcement officers in the same frame creates a nervous tension. It's frightening to see the imposing figures of the police present at the scene of lesbian lust. It's funny to see the dumbfounded police lined up like toy soldiers when confronted with lesbian desire.

A stylistically very different tape, *Safer Sex Slut* (1988), by Carol Leigh, features Leigh, a.k.a. Scarlot Harlot, dressed in a black bathing suit, leopard-skin jacket, dog collar, and a strand of pearls, performing a music video—a Janis Joplin-style anthem extolling the virtues of safe sex:

9. Ibid., p. 38.

> I won't become disease infected/Me I'll be so well protected/I always pay my income tax/I eat granola for my snack/I don't make fun of lumber jacks/Or mess with sheep that have anthrax/Safe sex/At the movies, in a car/In a bathroom, at a bar/Safe Sex.

The song's preposterous criteria of goodness and safety, renders the whole notion of a safe *sexuality* ridiculous, while boldly promoting the notion of practicing safe sex. At the same time, *Safe Sex Slut* employs humor to diffuse feelings of resentment that accompany condom use. Leigh proclaims, "The bedroom is the last frontier. Condoms leave a souvenir." Behind this song is the belief that there is no moral lesson to be learned from AIDS.

> The comic hero thrives by his vices. The tragic hero is destroyed by his virtue. Moral paradox is the crux of the drama.

In *Safe Sex Slut,* Leigh becomes the comic hero who survives by her vices. Her preoccupation with safety motivates her pursuit of pleasure. The two lesbians in *Keep Your Laws Off My Body* are heroes threatened because of their virtue. Moral paradox shapes the lives of queers: we are gay-bashed for living our lives honestly; we survive by celebrating the virtues for which we are despised.

[**Self-Mockery**]

"The things one takes seriously are one's weaknesses."

Yet another axiom in Ludlam's manifesto can be revisited in terms of a new, queer structure of feeling, reread in relation to AIDS-activist documentaries that only cast activists in a heroic light. A video that integrates performance and documentary, *Marta: Portrait of a Teenage Activist* (1990), by Mathew Ebert and Ryan Landry, exhibits the importance of this approach. Similar to Huff's *Rockville Is Burning,* and John Greyson's documentary on the sixth International AIDS Conference, *The World Is Sick (Sic)* (1989), the tape was shot during actual events—in this case, an ACT UP protest at the Centers for Disease Control in Atlanta. Dressed in very convincing parochial schoolgirl drag, Landry plays an overzealous, approval-seeking new member of ACT UP named Marta. Ebert taped the action, which was organized to protest the CDC's refusal to recognize lesbians as an epidemiological category in relation to AIDS, as well as to demonstrate against Georgia's sodomy laws, upheld in the infamous *Bowers v. Hardwick* Supreme Court decision. Ebert also conducted interviews with AIDS activists about Marta, using actual events to stage a fictional story that comments on the social dynamic of activism. Despite her annoying eagerness to please everyone, all the activists interviewed were fond of Marta.

The character Marta must have been named after the Atlanta public transportation system, also named MARTA. Additionally, the name brings to mind the word martyr. She is an overachiever—distributing hundreds of flyers advertising the upcoming actions under the doors of rooms at a motel occupied solely by activists who are there to attend the action. Marta holds her own protests. She demonstrates outside a theater in Atlanta presenting the movie *Peter Pan.* Underneath the marquee Marta screams into a bullhorn, "Why can't Peter Pan be played by a real fairy!? Shame! Shame! Stop Cathy Rigby! Stop Peter Pan! Now!"

"You are a living mockery of your own ideals. If not, you have set your ideals too low."

This Ludlam axiom expresses cynicism coupled with faith. Although it is true that queers are not martyrs by definition, the end many of us seek to achieve—liberation—is righteous. In *Marta* the profound sense of uncertainty that queer activists experience is presented as an important factor to be considered alongside the reasons that compel us to take action. Thus, the tape adapts the aims of Ridiculous Theater to the agenda of AIDS activism.

Landry and Ebert's insightful parody of the social behavior of activists, although witty and accurate in many respects, raises issues of sexism within queer structures of feeling. Although Landry's performance works as successful gender-fuck, why are issues of uncertainty played out solely through the actions of a female character? A similar question can be posed about *The World Is Sick (Sic)*. In that work, too, the main character is an inept woman played by a man in drag. In my experience, many women activists are seasoned organizers, and many are lesbians. They are not dizzy martyrs, nor are they uncertain about their political motives and beliefs. At the same time, both tapes exhibit a significant absence—uncertain, anxious gay men. It is not the drag performances per se that suggest sexism. In the practice of Ridiculous Theater the drag queen "poses the problem of psychosexual identity: to what extent male and female conduct, masculinity and femininity, are social role identities, cultural artifacts, what they are, might be, should be—how valid these roles are, how natural."[10] In these two examples, the drag performances share these aims; however, they function to the exclusion of male characters working through the fears and ambivalences we all have toward engaging in political actions. In both videos, this absence becomes manifest as a displacement of all negative feelings onto the female protagonists.

10. Ibid., p. 54.

[Ridiculous versus Lyrical]

In contrast, uncertainties and insecurities produced by the AIDS crisis constitute the fabric of Tom Kalin's *They Are Lost to Vision Altogether* (1988). No conclusion can be drawn from the tape, yet it produces powerful emotional effects—sadness and an almost overwhelming sense of loss. Fragments of many different texts—visual and aural, stolen from movies and television—as well as original images produced by Kalin are interwoven in ways that produce confusion. Material from the nightly news collides with images from porn; dialogue from Hollywood films underscores archival footage. Rapid editing and music propel the viewer from one section to another. The structure of this tape has much in common with a play written by Ludlam, who described Ridiculous Theater as "a bundle of series of intensive image explosions."[11] Like Ludlam, Kalin refuses a claim to original authorship, but in one respect his tape differs markedly from Ridiculous Theater. Its power rests in the evocative material Kalin has collaged, and it relies on the sentimentality of the images. *They Are Lost to Vision Altogether* is lyrical; Ridiculous Theater is never lyrical.

The elegiac qualities of Kalin's tape express feelings of loss and absence many of us experience as the cumulative effect of many deaths from AIDS. We watch what is all around us turn into memory. We talk about an ever-increasing number of people in the past tense. We experience nostalgia for events that happened, not years ago, but months ago, weeks ago, because we miss people who participated in these events and died shortly after. To watch videos about AIDS activism produced two or three years ago, those of us who have been involved in the movement must be prepared

11. Ibid., p. 44.

to encounter the faces of at least twenty people who are now dead. Many of us are in a perpetual state of mourning.

This was not so merely ten, fifteen, twenty years ago. A very different worldview reigned when Ludlam conceived his theater. Ridiculous Theater represented a radical attempt, calculated to call into question the dominant moral order constitutive of the dominant social order—to reveal our socially formed identities to be characterological lies. In the words of Stefan Brecht, it "approaches the effects if not the status of a popular revolutionary art."[12] Ridiculous Theater "considers established and recognized conventions of its medium as part of the culture's technique for artists and costumers to escape authentic actuality, and therefore would allow the artist to employ them only in a destructive manner—i.e., destroying the effect of tranquilized impersonality—hence insists on sabotage—of effects—at all points."[13]

Ridiculous Theater questioned notions of sincerity, authenticity, and truth. AIDS activists also need to question sincerity, authenticity, and truth, but, unlike Ridiculous Theater, AIDS activist videos cannot sabotage all emotional effects. Ultimately we die, and the U.S. government does nothing. The situation is obscene. It's ridiculous. The effect provokes laughter—the kind of laughter that forces tears and hurts the stomach, laughter filled with rage. For Ludlam, "What was funny was evident: the ridiculous obscenity of the human race."[14]

"Evolution is a conscious process."

Throughout the development of this article I have felt as if I were writing polemically against death, a ridiculous endeavor. But a reasonable expectation can be derived from this preposterous refusal to accept death:

12. Ibid., p. 48.
13. Ibid., p. 83.
14. Ibid.

I refuse to accept the death of certain ideas and certain practices. The recent deaths of such great artists as Ludlam, Jack Smith, and Ethyl Eichelberger pose a challenge to all of us who accepted the death of the author as a condition of cultural criticism.[15] Ludlam's work was the product of a particular culture—gay culture, which is, in turn, the cumulative result of work done by and for a particular group of people, gay people—at a particular time in a particular place. His work is not lost with his death. Rather, the contributions of a figure like Ludlam can be measured by the different manifestations of his ideas in culture over time. The ridiculous is a tendency within queer structures of feeling, and its resonances are perceptible in the most recent emergence of queer art in all forms. And the ridiculous will continue to appear in different forms, despite the many deaths of those who have struggled to keep a queer culture of dissent alive.

15. Roland Barthes's argument concerning the "death of the author" meant to displace the hegemony of an author's intention underlying a text's meaning. The actual death of many great artists during the AIDS crisis reinvigorated the attention paid to the author–artist's role in art. I never rejected Barthes's contention that texts have many authors, including its readers, but AIDS compelled me to recognize the contributions of singular figures.

Operative Assumptions

4

Originally published as "Operative Assumptions," in *Resolutions: Contemporary Video Practices,* eds. Michael Renov and Erika Suderberg (Minneapolis and London: University of Minnesota Press, 1996), pp. 173–184. Minor revisions have been made for consistency.

THIS TEXT WAS WRITTEN IN THE EARLY NINETIES *before I completed my movie* Fast Trip, Long Drop. Fast Trip, Long Drop *was intended to be a summation of eight years of practice as a media activist. It was a kind of liquidation sale. "Everything," I thought, "must go." Before I could make a video that summarized a long period of activity, I needed to inventory and critically review the operative theoretical assumptions underlying my practice. "Operative Assumptions" follows the model of reflection and assessment established by "Picture a Coalition." It is no less prescriptive, but by the time I sat down to write "Operative Assumptions," my temperament had shifted. The unbridled enthusiasm—fueled by rage—that produced the call to action at the end of "Picture a Coalition" had been transformed by disappointment and fatigue into something more thoughtful and introspective. In this text and the video that followed (*Fast Trip*), I allowed doubt and uncertainty each to have a voice. The concluding essay of this collection, "More Operative Assumptions" continues this thread.*

You are a living mockery of your own ideals. If not, you have set your ideals too low. —*Charles Ludlam*[1]

Chapter 4 *Operative Assumptions*

For the past five years I have worked as a videomaker for the Gay Men's Health Crisis (GMHC) where I have been the coproducer, with Jean Carlomusto, of the "Living with AIDS" cable show, as well as the producer of many videotapes addressing the concerns of people living with HIV.[2] 71

In 1985, I started making video as a young artist searching for ways to represent the manifold processes through which people come into being

1. Charles Ludlam, "Manifesto: Ridiculous Theater, Scourge of Human Folly," in *The Complete Plays of Charles Ludlam* (New York: Harper and Row, 1989), p. vii.
2. The Gay Men's Health Crisis is the nation's oldest and largest AIDS service organization, providing services and advocacy to people with AIDS. *Living with AIDS* was

as subjects. I realized that by making video I could introduce the element of time into my work in ways I couldn't possibly achieve by making static images or installations. I wanted to represent the formation of subjectivities by creating conflicts between sound and image over time. Video seemed to be the most effective medium to picture the ways representations assign us places from which to identify. I was excited by its counter-hegemonic potential. Additionally, video was relatively cheap and I had access to equipment. It was easy to learn how to use.

As a student I began to question the ways video art had been canonized within art world institutions. In general, video made for galleries and museums pursued two tendencies. The first was a preoccupation with the formal limits of the medium; the other used the medium as a means to further the concerns of performance art. There were exceptions. Dara Birnbaum's work addressed issues of representation in video by appropriating and questioning network television. I have in mind Birnbaum's 1978 video *Technology/Transformation: Wonder Woman,* which repeated an image appropriated from a popular weekly television show of the superheroine transforming from a mild-mannered woman into Wonder Woman, spinning in circles and exploding. For me, this video rendered open the possibilities of a critical video practice.

Around the same time I was introduced to the works and writings of Martha Rosler and Dan Graham—two distinctly different artists who both used video to interrogate mass culture. Rosler's *Global Taste: A Meal in Three Courses,* a video installation at the New Museum in New York in 1985, was a fragmented collage of material presented on three monitors housed within a structure that did not permit the viewer to see all the monitors at the same time from any one vantage. The "interlocking motifs in

a weekly cable program produced by GMHC addressing concerns of people with AIDS and those who care for them.

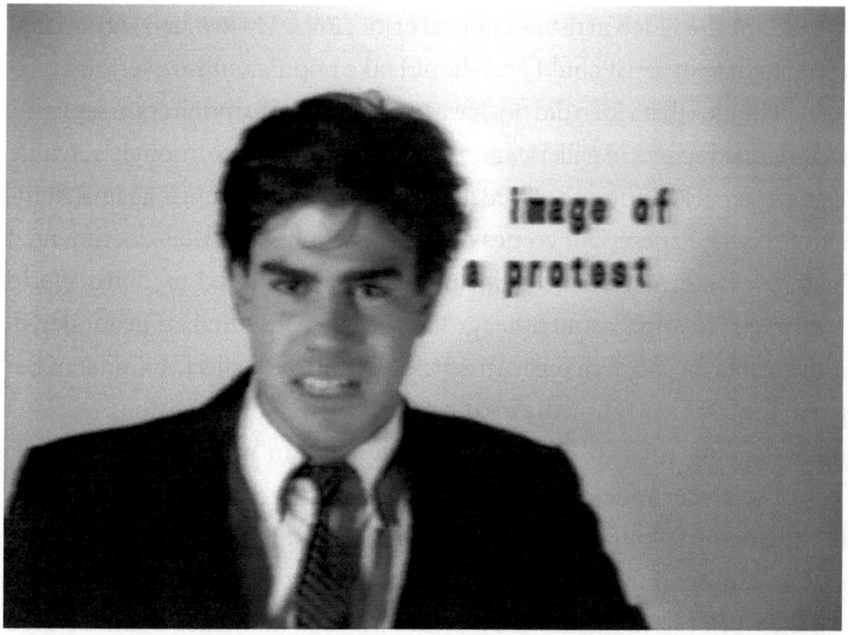

Figure 4.1 Gregg Bordowitz, *. . . some aspect of a shared lifestyle . . .*, 1986.

its videotapes are children, food, commercials and learning." The theme of the installation was "colonization of the self and of other countries, by media and advertising."[3] As a student, I was overwhelmed by the complexity of the work and its ambition to map complex social forces. Rosler's printed works, specifically, *The Bowery in Two Inadequate Descriptive Systems,* introduced me to criticism of left-identified documentary practices.[4]

Dan Graham's video *Rock My Religion* (1984–1985) introduced me to the idea of the video artist as cultural critic. *Rock My Religion* legitimated the idea that an artist could and should take popular culture seriously.

The idea that video did not have to be relegated to monitors in separate, well-defined spaces in galleries and museums came to me through watching Paper Tiger Television as it waged its own weekly cable struggle against dominant media. Paper Tiger comes out of a recent but not well-documented history of alternative media, including but not limited to Third World Newsreel, Videofreex, and other groups of alternative makers grounded in movements for social change. An article by Dee Dee Halleck, founder of Paper Tiger, "Some Arguments for the Appropriation of Television," inspired me at the same time I began to think of myself as an "activist videomaker."[5]

I was very much influenced by these producers for many reasons, but the one attribute they shared was an interest in using video, both inside and, more important, outside the context of galleries and museums. All the work I have mentioned fostered the idea that video could be used as a means to organize audiences around critical activities that challenge

3. Martha Rosler, "Global Taste: A Meal in Three Courses," gallery statement for "The Art of Memory: The Loss of History" (New York: New Museum of Contemporary Art, 1985).
4. Martha Rosler, "The Bowery in Two Inadequate Descriptive Systems," in *Martha Rosler: Three Works,* Nova Scotia Pamphlets 1 (Halifax: Press of the Nova Scotia School of Art and Design, 1981), pp. 11–57.
5. Dee Dee Halleck, "A Few Arguments for the Appropriation of Television," *High Performance* 37 (1987): 38–44.

the culture industry. The artists considered viewers to be participants in a process of making meaning. In formulating my own work I began to think of critical pedagogy as an ideal practice.

I think many video artists were and continue to be daunted by the monolithic enterprise of broadcast television. Artists feel that they can't possibly compete because of a lack of resources and access to broadcast venues. Video can be, and often is, employed in installation work to address conditions of spectatorship in the gallery or the museum. I can't limit myself to using video in this way. The broadcast dimension of television is the fundamental component of the medium. I am much more interested in television's broadcast capacity than in the multichannel video installation. I am interested in exploiting television's potential as an organizing tool. Further, I view broadcast television as a field within which to intervene and bring about meaningful change.

Commercial television is produced with an agenda: to dominate the leisure time of its audience in order to sell products, to engender a public of consumers. Fundamentally opposed to this, I have attempted to travel the way of Bertolt Brecht: to employ forms of entertainment that engage the critical skills of an audience, galvanizing the potential for collective action. I approach television production as an activist, employing video as a means of organizing. My work is a hybrid of concerns derived from critical theory affecting my own conditions of existence. I place my own subjectivity at risk within my work, drawing on my own daily experiences, using my own identity and the various subject positions comprising it. My interest in videomaking developed at the same time that I was coming out as a gay man and coming to consciousness about the AIDS epidemic. My first video, . . . *some aspect of a shared lifestyle* . . . (1986), considered the topic of the emerging AIDS epidemic in view of my concerns about the formation of subjectivity. It's a raw tape, juxtaposing first-person narration with varying medical opinions and differing representations culled from the dominant media—news reports, television specials, magazine and newspaper articles. While making this tape, I realized that I was part of an emerging identity. The AIDS crisis precipitated the formation of a new subjectivity—the person living with AIDS—a subject with a disease asserting his or her right to determine the conditions of his or her own health care. The formation of this identity was significant. People with a disease organized as a constituency, a political identity, questioning the ways they are positioned by authority and subjugated within the dominant culture. After the first tape, I became involved with the emerging AIDS activist movement, participating in several AIDS activist video collectives—Testing the Limits and DIVA TV (Damn Interfering Video Activists)—and producing television for GMHC. I tested positive for HIV antibodies in 1988; this informed my decision to make tapes by and for people living with HIV.

Over the past six years of AIDS activist television production I have come up with a set of fundamental organizing principles. The following is a "manifesto" to which I have added explanatory notes. I hesitate to use the word *manifesto.* This text lacks the force of certainty that often justifies the use of the term: it's riddled with ambivalences and ambiguities. In spite of these, I use the term. The following principles are intended to foster the spread of participatory democratic forms of media production and reception.

[Operative Assumptions Concerning the Community-Based Production of Television]

Definitions

Two concepts shape my understanding of what I will repeatedly refer to as "dominant culture." The first is "hegemony," which Raymond Williams defined as "a more or less adequate organization and interconnectedness of otherwise separated and even disparate meanings, values, and practices, which it specifically incorporates in a significant culture and an effective social order."[6]

The second concept is "tradition," defined by Williams as follows: "For tradition is in practice the most evident expression of the dominant and hegemonic pressures and limits. It is always more than an inert historicized segment; indeed it is the most powerful practical means of incorporation. What we have to see is not 'a tradition' but a *selective tradition:* an intentionally selective version of a shaping past and a pre-shaped present, which is then powerfully operative in the process of social and cultural definition and identification."[7]

Dominant culture is culture produced in the interests of the current hegemony. Its material means of support come from sources with an interest in maintaining the status quo. These are the corporate and government interests that determine the content and form of newspapers, magazines, television, films, and so on. "Tradition" is the principle that upholds the sanctity of the forms and the values determining representations. Dominant culture borrows and steals from alternative cultures that are produced on the margins of societies by communities whose lives and experiences aren't accounted for within the current hegemony. The margins are a space for research and development of new ideas and methods of production not necessarily permitted within established fields. Dominant culture changes and grows, incorporating novel approaches developed on the margins. By doing this it simultaneously responds to historical change as it constructs

6. Raymond Williams, *Marxism and Literature* (Oxford and New York: Oxford University Press, 1977), p. 115.
7. Ibid.

it. Disenfranchised communities are forced by necessity to act on and intervene within dominant culture to get the recognition and resources necessary to their survival.

There is a distinct difference between the production of commercial television and the community-based production of television. The latter is produced by disenfranchised groups who are not recognized, or are recognized in limited ways, on dominant television. Community television is no less deserving of the label "television" than what is considered appropriate for broadcast. The fight is to expand the notion of television to include the kinds of production now assigned a place only at the margins of broadcast and production.

In this context, community must be understood as a shifting, horizontally expanding entity open to change and growth. Communities of the disenfranchised are formed through negation. Forces within the dominant culture construct differences among subjects and establish exclusive principles that govern group formation. Subjects excluded by these criteria identify with each other along the lines of differences that have been established within the dominant field. Identity formations arise among the disenfranchised as a means to speak in a society that has refused them the opportunities to represent themselves. Alliances among different disenfranchised groups create the possibilities of new communities that transgress constructed boundaries. New alliances and coalitions give rise to communities that promote social equity, dismantling the structures of power that have shaped dominant culture.

Two Challenges

1. Ask yourself, "What images would I like to see more of in the world?" Make them.

2. Face the representational problems of the day in ways that affect your daily life.

The most widely recognized problem among community producers is lack of access to the means of television production. Disenfranchised groups affected by AIDS have little access to the equipment necessary to produce programs addressing the concerns of their communities. Broadcast standard gear is beyond reach, but the increased availability of small-format consumer cameras has enabled television production by disenfranchised groups. Video activists have been organizing cooperatives and collectives to share the resources they have.

Programs that activists produce don't get network airtime. Alternative distribution networks have been established to get these works shown—cable broadcasts, organizational newsletters, and relations among AIDS service organizations are just some of the means used to distribute activist video. Many of the videos produced at GMHC, including videos produced for the *Living with AIDS* cable show, are available through the GMHC catalog of AIDS educational material distributed nationally to health care institutions and service providers. An excellent example of community education efforts that employ video is the "Seeing through AIDS" program in New York—an innovative mobile teaching event that uses alternative and activist video as a stimulus for training and discussions about AIDS in many different workplaces.[8]

The kinds of representations, or lack of representations, addressing disenfranchised subjects within the field of dominant media can be a primary motivation for making video work. Television legitimates the

8. "Seeing through AIDS" is organized through Media Network, which publishes a catalog of the videotapes used in the program.

experience of some subjects, and provides a witness to the current times for anyone willing, or able, to identify as a member of "the general public." "The general public" is a fiction established to organize consumers around purchasing products. Anyone who may not fit the image of what advertisers want television viewers to imagine as the kind of people who want a particular product is excluded from the field of representation. For example, people with AIDS and HIV infection are often invited to speak about some of their experiences on television, but they are never pictured speaking to members of the audience who may also be people with AIDS and HIV. It may be a long time (perhaps never) before we see public service announcements directly addressing people with AIDS in the audience of television.[9] No one wishes to be the subject of that address. The repressed

9. This text was written before the advent of protease inhibitors and the subsequent development of marketing strategies to directly advertise HIV medications to people with HIV. It is now common to encounter billboards and bus shelter advertisements showing "healthy" and "happy" people with AIDS enjoying the benefits of treatment. These ads, however, are not primarily produced in the interests of people with HIV. Though I and many others do greatly benefit from new treatments, the pharmaceutical industry advertising campaigns are developed in the interests of companies' profits. An unfortunate development is the pharmaceutical industries' increased participation in public treatment "education." The particular interests each company has in its own product always threatens to compromise the scientific objectivity good education demands.

The drug company advertising campaigns have come under much criticism for creating a false picture of living with AIDS. They tend to downplay side-effects and to glamorize living with AIDS as a lifestyle. Still, I must admit that seeing the ads in public spaces did excite me. The first time I saw one on a subway platform, I felt welcomed as a member of the "general public." I looked around at my fellow commuters wondering who else might have HIV. It figures that PWAs would become welcome members of the general public when expensive products emerged. We went from being an ostracized group to a marketing demographic. This move was complex. It was in part a result of our own activism and the subsequent participation in the drug approval process our activism won. No doubt, our efforts to fight the stigma associated with AIDS also played some role.

fact is that the many people living with HIV and AIDS don't have a choice. The production, distribution, and broadcasting of video work intended for an audience of people with AIDS and HIV, representing some of the complexities of living with HIV, creates opportunities toward the inclusion of groups affected by AIDS into the audiences of television.

Nine Operative Assumptions

1. *Video is a medium, but television is a situation.* Video describes a means of production, a specific technology. Television production engenders a set of relations among workers: producers, writers, camera operators, lighting designers, sound engineers, and so forth. It also engenders relations between makers and viewers.

2. *Don't trust technology.* Did you have a hand in its development? Is it developed in your interests? Take what you can use and use what you can take. Technology is designed within the context of social relations. Thus, relations of power and dominance inform all decisions concerning its design, use and implementation:

> We have now become used to a situation in which broadcasting is a major social institution, in which there is always a controversy but which, in its familiar form, seems to have been predestined by the technology. This predestination, however, when closely examined, proves to be no more than a set of particular decisions, in particular circumstances, which were then so widely if imperfectly ratified that it is now difficult to see them as decisions rather than as [retrospectively] inevitable results.
>
> Thus, if seen only in hindsight, broadcasting can be diagnosed as a new and powerful form of social integration and control. Many

of its main uses can be seen as socially, commercially and at times politically manipulative.[10]

3. Television can be used in directed pragmatic ways *as a means of defensive action.* Television is a form of intervention, interfering with the current social order. Television can be a crudely fashioned weapon, like a handful of nails bound by electrical tape thrown at a group of armed soldiers. It can be a form of sabotage, like a wrench thrown into the works of an engine, or like a virus introduced into a computer system.

4. Television should not be limited to a means of defense. It can be proactive. Make television in the interests of community. This is the spiritual dimension of production. It requires faith. Have faith in the power of collective action and document the efforts of many different people working together toward common goals. Enfranchisement is the primary goal. The most significant feature of television production is its capacity to create opportunities for the formation of new audiences and communities.

I have seen groups of people accomplish great tasks through collective efforts—for example, the ACT UP, ACT NOW nonviolent takeover of the Food and Drug Administration in October 1988, and subsequent New York ACT UP actions at New York City Hall, the New York State Capitol, Saint Patrick's Cathedral, and so on. I have witnessed and documented all these actions.

5. On dominant television, images, words, and ideas seemingly have no causal relation to each other; and there are no beginnings or ends. Domi-

10. Raymond Williams, *Television: Technology and Cultural Form* (New York: Schocken Books, 1975), p. 23.

nant television presents itself as an immanent domain. There is no outside to dominant television. Television necessarily refers to itself to establish its own veracity. Exclusions and marginalizations figure within the field of the dominant as signifying absences that play a determining role regarding the choice of subject matter on television.

6. In community television production the ends are the means because new possibilities emerge when the means of production are in the hands of a self-determining group of people representing themselves. A community creates itself as it represents itself. Videomaking can foster a process of consensus building and can provide the arena in which goals are identified by a group.

7. Ontology and tactics merge on the television screen. The subjective conditions of the makers must be acknowledged as a fundamental factor informing all productions, broadcasts, and screenings. Static, the hissing, grainy emission of light and sound present on the screen of an operating television, is the presence of nothing—the positive, substantive form of nothingness. That we produce television at all is an attempt to cope with the existence of this static state. I realize that this may sound pretentious, but I think it's necessary to recognize the existential dimension of production, to state what is fundamentally at stake for the individual maker.

Two fundamental dialectical formulations structure my understanding of the contradictions inherent in making television. (1) I accept as a given fact that the dialectic between eros and thanatos is a determining factor affecting our actions. A dynamic tension exists between desire and death—the strong impulse toward the experiences of pleasure that disclose one's being to oneself exist alongside strong impulses toward the self-negation of one's being. The knowledge that one may die gives life its value. (2) I accept as a given fact the existentialist dialectic between being and nothingness. The agency of the subject is opposed by the arbitrary nature of the sign—when I speak I risk being understood in very different ways than I intended; perhaps I will not be understood at all. Meaning is always threatened by nonsense. Reason is always humbled by contingency. There are forces at work beyond one's control that can thwart one's best devised plans.[11]

To avoid facile, vulgar, deterministic accounts of events one must admit that there are limits to what one can know. All accounts must allow for unknown factors. No single cause can explain a situation. No explanation can sum up the totality of a situation. Truth, like tradition, is an absolute category established in the interests of an established order. Work that questions the status of truth in representation runs a great risk of exclusion from dominant media, but it serves the interests of those whose history has been done great violence by the official record.

11. The ideas of Andre Green have recently informed my thinking about how nothingness has substance. Green draws a distinction between nothing and no-thing. The origin of no-thing—which can be described as the presence of a structuring absence—is the missing maternal body. The ruptures in time produced by a mother's coming and going create a space for symbolization, as the infant forms an idea of the mother to hold onto while she is absent. This account of what Green terms "the negative" is an appropriate supplement to the formulations of section 7. My experience of television static as a "positive substantive form of nothingness"—a locution I believe I cribbed from Lacan—stems from a maternal relation I formed with the television set as a child. I have always sought the comfort of television. It addresses me and places me; it's always available; it continues without me when I turn it off, and it always reappears when I turn it on.

For more about Green's ideas "on the work of the negative" in psychoanalysis see Andre Green, *Andre Green at the Squiggle Foundation,* ed. Jan Abram (London and New York: Karnac Books, 2002).

8. Television cannot instrumentally affect the actions of viewers. Television presents options and possibilities for action. Community producers can picture forgotten options and ignored possibilities.

9. Television doesn't belong to the producer. The producer is not its sole reason for being. Any spectator can and should claim part ownership of television's production.

Nagging Afterthoughts

1. The issue of whether to make video or film is not only an issue of medium. It can be framed as an issue of idiom. Choosing between video production and film production is often framed as an economic decision by many producers. Videos are cheaper to produce, but films—because of their greater production values—circulate in ways that exclude video. Film festivals and movie theaters don't show ambitious video works, regardless of the productions' cultural importance. This division in status is changing. In general, the distinctions between the two media are breaking down. Most broadcast television is filmed in production and many films are now edited on videotape.

Neither television nor cinema are pure categories anymore. Accepting that as a given, I am committed to making television. I produce video work that draws on, refers to, and comments on the history of television.[12]

12. This argument seems to contradict claims I've made elsewhere crediting the influence of filmmakers—like Yvonne Rainer—as central to my work. There's no contradiction here. In this text I emphasized the decision behind video production over filmmaking, because there was much debate about the status of medium when I wrote this. I wanted to make work as formally engaging and ambitious as Rainer's using video rather than film; my attachment to the medium derived from my history with television grafted onto the emerging technical possibilities available through con-

The decision to make television is a choice to produce within and improve on a set of idioms within a specific history of production. I like television because it is cheap, fast, superficial, and disposable—like a daily newspaper. To make film is to work within the idioms of cinema. A decision to work within either category is founded on the belief that there are still tendencies within each worthy of pursuit.

2. *The category of experimental work in video has been challenged and broadened over the past decade.* The relation between the speaking subject and the subject of address is being reconsidered from fresh perspectives. The structure and formation of identity is being questioned with new rigor. Addressing new audiences, communities, and constituencies is the goal of much new work. Even more ambitious is current video work that attempts to form new constituencies by picturing alliances among disenfranchised groups.

There has been a shift away from previous areas of experimentation. The limits of the video medium and the science behind television have been thoroughly explored by artists like Nam June Paik who strongly identify with the notion of the avant-garde and whose concerns were formed out of formalist problems rooted in the history of painting and sculpture. Video has already been used effectively in galleries to defy viewers' assumptions about fixed notions of time and space. Dan Graham, Vito Acconci, Bruce Nauman, and many others have challenged the spectator's trust in the bodies' sense of presence and continuity. The status of truth in documentation has been questioned and dealt serious blows by artists

sumer access to video equipment. Even at the time of writing, I included movies among my influences, both popular and art films. Some of the films that most inspired me—though certainly not all—I saw on television and video.

mentioned before—Rosler and Paper Tiger Television. Godard and others associated with cinema have made their contributions by posing tough philosophical questions about television.

Many contemporary videomakers start from a critical interrogation of dominant television, developing complex, rich, and affirming representations of disenfranchised subjects and communities—*Tongues Untied* by Marlon Riggs or *L Is for the Way You Look* by Jean Carlomusto.

In general, significant shifts have occurred in theoretical conceptions of audience. The notion of an audience composed of artists and videomakers has been under assault for the past two decades. In the eighties, under the Reagan presidency, decreases in arts funding and conservative attempts at censorship have limited the resources of arts institutions and provoked competition among artists. Republican policies have also politically charged the atmosphere, resulting in a resurgence of identity politics. My work is the product of these times. The AIDS crisis created a situation in which my identity as an artist became subordinate to my identity as an activist, although making video has remained my primary activity.

[**Critique of Previous Work in View of My Experiences and Thoughts on the Future**]

In the spring of 1988, within two months, I tested HIV-antibody-positive, came out to my parents as gay, and decided to seek help concerning my alcohol and drug use. This was the densest moment of my life. Since then I have come to realize that there is no reason why I'm HIV-positive, why some people get sick and why some people die. Although there are historical conditions that explain the crisis, there is no reason behind AIDS. But there is meaning. My experiences are rich with meaning. They're full of pain, irony, and hope.

The work I've done in the past few years was predicated on the conviction that action must be taken toward ending government inaction on the AIDS epidemic. This conviction led me to a representational practice with a set of pragmatic goals. This work was often limited to performing a specific function: the documentation of the 1988 nonviolent takeover of the Food and Drug Administration, the provision of vital information concerning alternative medical treatments for HIV-antibody-positive people, safer-sex educational videos for bars and theaters. There is some amount of certainty behind the production of this work. Positions must be stated clearly and asserted authoritatively, leaving little room for speculation. Fear of death often goes unacknowledged in much AIDS activist videos. Sexual identities are often presented unproblematically. Safer-sex educational materials often don't consider the complexities of desire.[13]

I still hold the same convictions that motivated me, but now there is also a need for video work that explores the subjectivity of a person living with HIV infection. The documentary form predominates AIDS and HIV media. I've contributed to the development of this corpus. Now I think it is important to grapple with the subjective conditions of living with HIV in ways that challenge conventional means of representation. We must consider the uncertainties inherent in the experience of being a person with HIV, uncertainties regarding sexuality, agency, and death.

The AIDS epidemic calls all previous notions of sexual identity into question because the epidemic necessitates talking about sexual behavior

13. For more detailed information about GMHC safer-sex educational videos see: "Do It! Safer Sex Porn for Girls and Boys Comes of Age," by Jean Carlomusto and Gregg Bordowitz, in *A Leap in the Dark: AIDS, Art, and Contemporary Cultures,* eds. Allan Klusacek and Ken Morrison (Toronto and Buffalo: Vehicle Press, 1992), pp. 177–183.

rather than identity. For example, new categories such as "men who have sex with other men" were developed in the field of sex education to account for the many men who do not identify themselves as "gay." Now, as the lesbian and gay liberation movement enters a new decade, new ideas about identities and alliances are being considered among lesbians and gay men. Established identities are being questioned. Media artists now have to recognize the fragility and historical specificity of identities. The shifting forces that shape identity during the AIDS crisis must be named and studied.

Also, new work about AIDS must question agency, the role of the individual in social change. The AIDS activist movement has posed a significant threat to the dominant order. It has been a catalyst for a growing health care movement in the United States. People with AIDS and HIV have been cast as agents of change in a number of intersecting fields, such as medicine, law, government, and business. Our struggle raises fundamental issues concerning people's rights of choice to control their own bodies. We have called into question long-held assumptions about government's sovereignty over matters of life and death.

People with AIDS and HIV must conduct their lives in the face of death because no person with HIV knows if or when she or he may get sick or die. Activists rarely see concrete results from their efforts, yet they continue to struggle. Work that addresses these issues will radically change current thinking about representation and AIDS.

Personal records and testimonies are valuable additions to the growing body of work that is shaping the ways the AIDS epidemic affects our lives. They are part of efforts to legitimate the concerns of people hardest hit by the AIDS epidemic and to pressure established institutions to take responsibility for some of the work that needs to be done in facing the continuing crisis. New video work that explores the psychic complexities of living with HIV can bring an acute awareness of mortality into debate with the ordinary tasks of daily existence. I have started a new series of portraits in video of people living with HIV. They are going to be a regular feature on the *Living with AIDS* cable program. I've completed six so far and would like to make as many as fifty.[14] The first five portraits are two to five minutes in length. Each features a subject who looks directly into the camera and identifies as a person living with HIV. Then the subject is pictured in a variety of settings—the home, the office, a restaurant—talking about a variety of topics, not necessarily about HIV. However, once the subject discloses his HIV status, whatever follows in the video—a walk down the street, a game of pool, a discussion about pets—becomes a metaphor for living with AIDS or HIV. I am interested in exploring this. Perhaps, new ways of discussing mortality can develop out of this effort. In the portraits, I'm trying to reconcile an acute awareness of mortality with the monotony of daily life.

There has been a shift in the focus of this text that exemplifies a shift in my thinking about video work concerning AIDS. The first part of this text is an attempt to sum up aspects of community television paying special attention to pragmatic concerns. These ideas were formulated at a time when AIDS activist video was not yet an identifiable body of work, as it is today. When they were developed, I was motivated by the need for progressive cultural work about AIDS and I gave much thought and energy to fostering its existence. With the establishment of this small but visible category of video, new questions arise concerning the representation of AIDS, so I have recently become preoccupied with more subtle and complex questions about illness and death, issues that capture my attention for the obvious reason: my own HIV infection.

14. Since I wrote this article I continued to make portraits of people with HIV and expanded the project to include advocates who aren't positive. There are about fifteen portraits now. I make them as sketches or for specific use in fund-raising efforts.

Sometimes I question whether or not I should continue making work about AIDS. I feel trapped by my infection. My work and the scope of my interests often seem reduced to the disease. Yet, I can't exclude AIDS and HIV from the frame of my thinking. It has become a prism through which I view the world, and I expect that it will unfortunately take up more space on the horizon of my future.

[An Internal Dialogue]

Currently, I'm at work on an hour-long video concerning the problem of remaining hopeful in the face of increasing loss and despair.[15] It attempts to picture the rage and sense of futility many people with AIDS or HIV experience. I feel a great sense of urgency motivating me to make the tape. Much is at stake.

Sometimes the forces motivating one to make work are not easily located in an identification with a cause external to and greater than the subject making the work—a movement, a group, an audience. Sometimes one has no conscious understanding of why one is making the work. Am I regressing into some kind of expressionist position mystifying the creative process? As a student, I made a commitment against any mystifying practices assigning privilege to an author, a figure, a signature, a gesture. I resisted the notion of the artist as a lonely alienated soul who is the bearer of a unique mark, the product of his individuality, a testament to the universal and transcendent nature of the human spirit. I formed some early assumptions behind my work arguing against neoexpressionism and the "return" to "traditional values" that was taking over the art world during

15. I was referring to the video *Fast Trip, Long Drop,* which was then beginning to take shape in my mind.

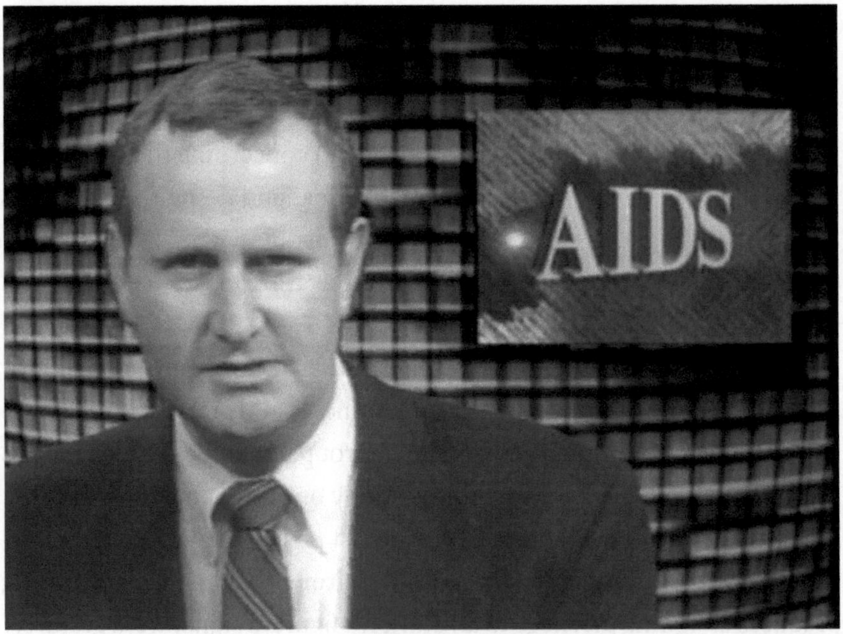

Figure 4.2 Gregg Bordowitz, *Fast Trip, Long Drop*, 1993.

the first years of the Reagan revolution. My peers and I vigorously opposed this tendency. These were the formative circumstances of my education as an artist. They continue to inform the decisions I make today.

Has my opposition to some formulations of expressionism enabled me to ignore the presence of my own unconscious? Has it limited my ability to understand the role of my unconscious? There have been times in the recent past when I repressed my own ambivalences in order to convey a sense of certainty in my activist work. When I was most intensely involved in AIDS activist politics, I was unable to admit any sense of doubt in my work. Doubt, uncertainty, and contingency were temporarily removed from my vocabulary. This was not a crime. I feel more curious than guilty reflecting on the limits of previous efforts. Circumstances seemed to demand it, and now I understand why. It was necessary for me to focus on the problems of representation concerning people with AIDS in general rather than become mired in the circumstances of my own infection—the arena in which I experience fear about the future. This was a good but inefficient means of coping. It left much unattended. Now, I must pose new questions and maybe formulate some answers.

The more rules I try to establish, the more questions arise. Every time I formulate a principle, I feel burdened by the demand to locate its origin of thought. Every assumption is founded on a previously established received idea. My thinking is a rickety structure that can barely support the weight of surrounding circumstances. I call it home.

5

Boat Trip

Originally published as "Boat Trip," *American Imago* 51, no. 1 (spring 1994): 105–125. Minor revisions have been made for consistency.

THIS TEXT RECORDS A VACATION I TOOK *with the other members of my HIV support group: David Barr, Spencer Cox, Mark Harrington, Derek Link, and Peter Staley. The group was self-run. For seven years, we met every other week, taking turns hosting the meetings at our homes. In the meetings, we took turns talking about whatever issues we needed to address, and for as long as we needed. The group was an extraordinary example of self-care emerging out of the democratic principles and methods of our activism. In those days, it seemed as if we were organized to deal with everything. If a friend fell ill, an efficient care team quickly pulled together. Schedules for around-the-clock nursing were established. We formed our support group to address our fears about death and to lay the groundwork for the future when each of us would die. All the members of the group are still alive.*

[11/10/92 British Virgin Islands]

On the beach at Peter Island. Having trouble with the new equipment. Short circuit in the steady-cam. Waterproof camera is awkward. It limits the remote control function to the zoom, and the autofocus in the camera doesn't easily focus. These problems frustrate me. I have great hopes for the trip and its video documentation. What do I want from the trip? The video? The compelling factor behind it all, the reason we're here together: we are all HIV-positive. That's why we formed the support group two years ago. Six gay HIV-positive men who do AIDS work full-time.

I expect an answer at the end of this trip and I expect to capture it on video. An answer to what? Why? There's no answer. It's a flawed inquiry. A poorly stated, ignorant question. To ask is to posit reason. There's no reason why we're all positive. Must abandon this line of questioning. I know that. I'll drive myself crazy asking. I must be resigned to whatever I come away with. Is it possible to separate the event from its documentation? The documentation is coextensive with the event. Once the event is over the record becomes an entity in and of itself, bearing a lessening relation to the actual event. Let the experience dictate the record, if I can. It seems as though I once privileged experience over thought. I was open to much more than I am now. Now I want to be able to predict the outcome of experience, know it, order it, and guard myself from the unknown. The unknown could mean death. It is uncertain that the trip will yield anything more than the pleasure of vacation. Perhaps, deepening relationships among us. Is that enough?

The onset of the trip is burdened with the memory of significant events. This November 9, 9:20 A.M. is the second year anniversary of Ray's death.[1] At that moment, I find myself on a plane with five other infected men sharing a vacation trying to have a good time before inevitably one or more of us becomes ill. It felt appropriate that the date of the group's departure was the anniversary of Ray's death. As though this date and the distance from the event marked a new line of flight toward something living rather than away from something dead. November 9 is also the anniver-

1. Ray Navarro (1964–1990) was a major figure in ACT UP and talented videomaker who cofounded DIVA TV. He was also my very dear friend. His death, a profound experience for me, is a recurring theme in this book.

sary of Kristallnacht. I am aware of this as I am aware of my mortality. Forces of evil conspire against me and my kind. I feel threatened. Conflicted. I also feel reborn. This sailing trip holds the promise of renewal. I want to live. It's very difficult to admit that. Superstitious. Someone's going to take it all away from me if I don't keep quiet. Just pretend you're not enjoying yourself and no one will try to spoil your fun. I'll survive if I pretend to be miserable. Fondness for misery. Must stop.

Last night on the boat we all fell asleep early. The two plane trips and bus ride getting here were tiring. Fell asleep at 7:00 P.M. on deck. At some point I woke up and went below. The rocking of the boat awakened me periodically and I restlessly alternated between deck and bunk. It's beautiful here. Fresh dense green covering jagged rock islands floating on clear green fields; the water changing hue with shifts in current, changes in depth. On the first night, at sunset, both the sun and the moon are for a moment present in the sky, diametrically opposed as though one implies the other; one is the reflection of the other; one is the projection of the other; one is the absence of the other.

I slept next to Peter part of the night. He is a good little scout. It's his father's boat, *Tucket Mist.* He has sailed these waters many times. First with his family as a child and now as the captain leading his band on this expedition. None of us, except Peter, has ever sailed before.

This first day, we all took off our shirts revealing ourselves to the setting sun. Mark, Spencer, and I have similar rashes. My doctor told me that the rash on my arms and back is caused by my infection. I never believed that HIV was the cause, until now. The fact that each of us is infected with the same kind of virus is astonishing. My awareness of this fact is unconsciously mediated, managed, so that the full emotional weight doesn't register. I feel embarrassment when my denial is momentarily revealed to me. The sad reason for our group's existence is made present to my mind. I wonder if we will transcend this, if our union will be justified by something more than each individual's need for support. Our love for each other, perhaps. The horror of our common fate does not overwhelm me. We are here in spite of it, taking pleasure.

[**11/11/92**]

Yesterday, late in the day, I was able to get the steady-cam to operate. Shot good video. Made some nice images of the guys sailing and playing cards. Many familiar feelings are evoked hanging around with this group of men. I feel as if I've been in the company of these men all my life. They are my older male relatives who remain at the table after the women have removed the dinner dishes. They are the group of buddies passing joints in parked cars overlooking scenic points. Spending time with the support group reminds me most of my teenage years. Now, an adult, all my feelings are more on the surface, more available to me. I'm not stoned. I'm not repressing my affection for men. I still feel awkward at times. Must entertain them. Say smart things. Make them like me. I think they do. Immature.

Taking ddI,[2] Peter and I, together waiting to have coffee. Five more minutes. Everyone is waking up. Derek still sleeps. Today, we explore caves

2. Also known as Didanosine, ddI is a type of antiretroviral drug used to treat HIV. There are four forms of didanosine: chewable tablets, liquid, powder and capsules. The powder form must be added to water before it is swallowed. ddI should be taken on an empty stomach, at least thirty minutes before or two hours after eating. Side effects can include severe stomach pain, nausea, or vomiting; burning, numbness, or tingling in the hands, arms, feet, or legs; and vision problems. Other side effects may not be so serious and may lessen or disappear with continued use. Less serious side effects include diarrhea, upset stomach, headache, dizziness, anxiety, and sleep problems. For more information of ddI see "AIDSinfo: A service of the U.S. Department of Health and Human Services." Available at <http://aidsinfo.nih.gov/>.

and snorkel around a small island. Snorkeled yesterday for the first time ever. Scary. Will enjoy it more when I am accustomed to the floating sensation. I must have faith that I will not sink. Breathe through my mouth. We're all getting along well. I am getting closer to Peter. We have a flirtation. Must not take it too seriously.

Finished *To the Lighthouse.* A very different modernism from Joyce. (I read *Ulysses* a few months ago.) Woolf is more descriptive. More visual. Painterly. The writing is more joyous, less cynical than Joyce's. No parody. All the irony is contained within the point of view.

How should I describe my surroundings? I'm not very interested in doing it. The landscape is stunning. I'm preoccupied.

[**11/12/92**]

Yesterday turned out to be a long, fine day. Explored caves in the dinghy. Snorkeled coral reefs around and in between the Indians—a group of rocks jutting out of the water. Sailed for two, three hours to a heavily occupied cove. Conch fritters with pineapple juice in tourist restaurant. Hamburgers for dinner grilled on the boat. Attached a barbecue to the side rail, the common practice of the boats down here. At night, the coves are filled with boats moored for the night. A floating suburbia. Each has its own grill like a hearth. After dinner some of the guys played hearts below deck. David and I hung out together on deck talking under the stars. He started the group. He's its center, close friends with a number of us. Haven't seen each other in weeks. We needed to reconnect. Discussed everything: love, sex, friends, work.

We both focus on death in ways that interfere with our enjoyment of life, and we agreed that thinking about death all the time is a means to cope with anxiety. It makes us feel masterful, like we're on top of it all. Actually, the preoccupation prevents us from being present in the moment, enjoying experiences. Very difficult to overcome. We've very good reasons to be preoccupied with the possibilities of illness, death, and loss. At the moment when the conversation ran its course David summed it up, "I don't want to get sick." Stated simply. Matter of fact. For the record. I said, "I don't want you to get sick. I don't want to get sick. I don't want any of the others to get sick."

In the morning (11/11) on the dinghy, shot good video floating through the caves. Images of the guys, in snorkel gear, jumping off the boat. I think to myself that these are brave young men going to explore the unknown. Some of us were terrified to go snorkeling. I feared sharks. We all made jokes about *JAWS*. Floating over the fire coral I realized that I feel extremely vulnerable, fragile. Testing positive has made me very cautious. It can become suffocating and I must consciously resist the urge to protect myself from all uncertainty. I am young and, for the moment, healthy. I have some time.

Today we take mushrooms. Hallucinogens. Guys don't want me to tape this. I'll figure out a way to document it without interfering with their experiences.

Started to get anxious yesterday. The boat is smaller than it was in the beginning of the trip. A couple of times I wanted to snap at one of the shipmates. Can't remember why. I can sense the others feel the same way. I suggested that we have a group meeting. No one wanted to unpack his feelings in the middle of the trip. We decided that we'd have a group meeting on the last night, Sunday. Sounds good. I would like to do a group interview. Must ask the guys. (All agreed.)

[11/13/92]

Friday the 13th, we are struck by bad luck. The zipper on some mechanism affecting the sail has torn and we spend an hour trying to fix it unsuccessfully. Fortunately, the zipper does not affect the operation of the sail. It's just more difficult to unfurl and it doesn't fold neatly against the mast. Peter is greatly annoyed.

I'm tired. Didn't sleep well. Mosquitoes and rough waters conspired against me all night. Now I have a headache. Last night I smoked pot for the first time in five years. I'm curious about drugs again. I know I have "slipped." I don't feel terribly guilty. I didn't like it very much, and I've declined any subsequent turns on the many, many joints coming my way. Some of us are potheads. It was as I remembered it to be: difficult to breathe, self-conscious and paranoid. Unlike the past, I was able to manage all that and enjoy the pleasurable effects. The clouds took on mass. Colors brightened. I giggled. My desire for Peter increased. I wanted to suck his cock. Couldn't fall asleep last night with him naked next to me. Perhaps I will make my desires known to him. Risk: possible rejection. Awkward. No privacy on the boat. I'm horny. Haven't masturbated in days. The boat shrinks slowly. I would like to walk a great distance. Yesterday we sailed. I shot some video. Used the microphone to pick up fragments of chatter. Many jokes about yachting. Each of us did his imitation of Katharine Hepburn in *The Philadelphia Story*—"My, she was yar!"

We did not take the mushrooms on Thursday. Mark and Derek were ambivalent and convinced us to wait. The island we chose to spend the afternoon on was beautiful—palm trees, white sand, cacti and flowers, cliffs—but the sun was harsh and the shade under the palms housed mosquitoes and gnats. We all crowded under a lean-to that Peter erected using a sheet, two oars, and the dinghy. We huddled under this tropical wilderness shelter as though the serenity of the island was masking a violent storm. As a group we are thrown together by the threatening circumstances of the epidemic; we replicate this predicament wherever we gather.

This morning I was thrown out of the bed by the sensation of falling. I sat upright out of a deep sleep, saying aloud, "I'm falling." No one was around to hear me. I had been feeling crowded by the presence of the others, but waking up from this dream of an endless plunge, with no one lying next to me, I felt alone. Sad. I'm afraid of being thrown out of control by the drugs. Maybe I already am out of control and the desire to get high is a symptom. I feel guilty. I think of Richard. He was a junkie for seven years, clean now for ten. He appears to me as a fantasy figure, policing my desire to get high. I'm torn. I don't, at the moment, feel threatened. I don't want pot. I don't like it. I won't drink, but I want to take the mushrooms. I want to feel fully present. For a moment last night, high, looking at the stars with David, I felt like I was nowhere else. It's so rare that I'm not preoccupied with the nagging feeling of much unfinished business.

Relations among the crew are tense. I sense flashes of rage, but there have been no fights. Aggressive behavior manifests in competitive card playing, teasing and behind-the-back-quips. We'll be all right. We survived the worst yet today. No wind and then the sail dysfunction. No one got out of hand, and Peter kept his cool.

No video today. Too tired. Smoked pot last night and no sleep. Hard to concentrate now. So far, I've shot an hour and a half of tape. Enough for a nice short about the trip. A travelogue.

There will be no secrets at the end of this trip. No revelations. The most profound revelations I have are the repeated momentary realizations that there are no secrets, no prescriptions. The most important fact, the most fundamental thought, the most satisfying idea: all I have is the meaning of the moment. The feelings produced by the experience. Difficult to record. The effort is necessary. With video, writing, storytelling I'm holding on to the most valuable traces of experiences, the trace elements (mining metaphors come to mind), whether or not I successfully translate them for others to identify with. Who are these others?

Ate at a small restaurant called Sidney's Peace and Love. Small BBQ hut in a tiny cove. Approaching the dock in our dinghy a fat black man with large rough hands and larger hard worn bare feet grabs our rope and pulls each of us onto the dock—Sidney the proprietor. Approached by two black women who ask us, "Where are your women?" Peter replies, "we have no women." "We're not traveling with women." The women laugh long and hard. We are embarrassed. There are other white tourists. Guy-girl-guy-girl-guy-girl around long picnic tables, eating. I had chicken. Others had lobster and fish—snapper or grouper.

[11/15/92 Virgin Gorda. Sunday Morning.]

Yesterday was not splendid. Rained all day. Everything wet. Crew crowded into cabin below. Cards. Reading. Stagnant conversation. Some tense exchanges. Nothing irreparable. We all go to town, except for Mark. This town is a disgusting tourist trap designed to evoke nostalgia for colonialism.

Captain Peter is bitten from head to toe by mosquitoes. To add to his troubles the boat's starter has malfunctioned. Had to bring a mechanic out to the boat to take a look. A cute young blond Australian. The crew smiled, giggling when he went below to examine the engine. When he passed me, I looked skyward and batted my eyelashes—aware that Mark was watching me. It had the desired effect. Mark laughed out loud.

Dinner at an expensive restaurant—Drakes. Good food. I had lobster. Waitress flirted with me. I flirted back. Conversation among the guys was stale. Each gave his version of what went wrong with the AIDS movement. We've all had this conversation before. No one's point of view ever changes; each maintains his own version. I think that history has changed and the movement wasn't organized to tackle the larger issues of universal access to health care. Groups have internal limits and it is the nature of movements to shift, grow, and change. Permanent revolution. Peter thinks the demands to expand our focus were too great, resulting in bad faith among the activists. We should have established hierarchically organized protest groups with a core group of leaders rather than an anarchic participatory democracy. Mark thinks that a number of activists operating in bad faith auto-critiqued the movement to death; he agrees with David who is guardedly optimistic. David sees how the movement continues in the efforts of newly organized groups. In addition, he points out that many of us worked our way through the ranks and now occupy positions within the established mainstream organizations, where we can be more effective. Spencer agreed with some opinions, disagreed with others, his mind elsewhere, maybe thoughts of graduate school. Derek watches silently with a look on his face that I interpret as representing the fear, terror, and dread he experienced growing up in a cold family ignorant of his needs. I'm probably projecting these feelings onto his face. More likely, he's just as bored as everyone else with this chatter.

All went to bed early. David and I had a whispering conversation for a few moments before I went to my bunk below. He slept on deck. I told him that I was disappointed in the conversation. We are wasting valuable time not talking about the real issues which cause us pain. David responded that we have learned to play together on this trip; this should not be underestimated. When we're swimming, snorkeling, or playing cards, risks are taken and levels of intimacy are reached. He's right. I'm blind to almost all signs other than spoken words and stated affections.

We did not take the mushrooms on Saturday. It would have been awful. Perhaps, today, Sunday, the last day. Sun is shining and there's trouble. One of the battery ranks ran dead. They're not charging. Peter's a mess. We planned a large brunch, but David has just reported that the batter is burning because the pan and the stove are not right for each other. He abandoned the pancake project. Eggs and cereal.

Yesterday I shot some good images of Peter in a yellow slicker and white Calvin Klein briefs, scrubbing the deck in the pouring rain. He was "pleased" by the opportunity, in his words, "to use nature's forces to our advantage." I fear that he is the first to crack.

Finished *Been Down So Long, It Looks Like Up to Me.* Enjoyed it. A period piece. Dated, but I strongly identified with the protagonist who desperately tries to hold onto his "cool" throughout many trying situations that he gets himself into without seeing his own role in his fate. He consciously wages a battle to hold onto his "immunity," his "exemption" from mediocrity and responsibility. Peter Pan. The repeated use of the word "immunity" takes on a completely unintended use as I read this book. My HIV infection represents an enormous responsibility to me. I have to care for myself in ways I never imagined. It has made the transition to adulthood more painful than I think it would have been otherwise. The uncertainty the protagonist, Gnossos Papodoupolis, faces in his travels is the same uncertainty I face—mortality. His extreme fear of death drives his efforts to find romantic love. So does my own fear. For Gnossos, the fear is not manifest in the threat of illness. For him death comes in the form of conformity. I identify with that, being a child born of the sixties and its idealism. My idealism is fettered by the prospects of a limited future. An acute awareness of mortality has forced me to seek refuge in conformity. I seek stability more now than ever before. Are all twenty-eight-year-olds worried about who will care for them if they should get ill suddenly? I worry about not having a comfortable home to retire to when I get ill. Will I be able to live comfortably when I am bedridden? I seek the refuge offered by romantic love, though a relationship of that kind has not yet materialized. Part of the problem is that I'm waiting for it to materialize. Gnossos and I have much in common. We both feel rage about the loss of our youth. *I'm so young, so god damn young*—(Patti Smith singing "Privilege," a song I played as often as I could until some of the others on the boat screamed for a change in music). The threat of illness and death has spoiled my youth. I want to live to turn thirty. I want to grow old.

When I read on the inside cover of the dust jacket of *Been Down So Long* that the author, Richard Farina, died in a motorcycle accident two days after the book's publication, I knew that I must read it. As though my father, who died at thirty, had written it for me. Words of wisdom from the beyond. He's telling me to "keep onto your cool, man." "Oohbop shebam." Now, I will start Genet's *The Thief's Journal.* I strongly identify with Genet's existentialism. He writes poetry and erases it, writes it again and erases it again. Genet knows that one can only experience the presence of what is lost by losing it, over and over again. The meanings of my reading selections become apparent to me. I have just learned something about my relation to my lost father. I can only have his love if I fantasize about his death.

I've not accurately documented this trip. I'm collecting images and fragments, recording my thoughts, but I've failed to capture the day to day effort of leaving our worries behind. We never left them behind. For moments they were well hidden. Returning to our lives reveals them to us, renewed and vigorous. As if they had a rest, too. A vacation from us. I imagine a place where problems go to get away from our good spirits, where evil organizes its enterprise.

We have had some brief focused group conversations about living with HIV that quickly disintegrated. During one I expressed my resentment toward another support group brought together by some of our friends and lovers who are HIV-negative. This satellite group is organized around a similar mandate to our group: people who work in AIDS full-time and who have close relationships with people who are HIV-positive—us. I am annoyed that a group is organized to cope with our deaths. Of course, that's not the sole purpose of the group, but it is a primary concern. It all makes sense. Too much sense. We are too well organized. Prepared to face situations for which one can't possibly prepare. One can wait for death conscious of the waiting, or one can busy oneself with the minute details of daily tasks. Either way, one waits. It is easier to share the burden by waiting with others than it is to wait entirely alone. Certainly some portion of the burden must be borne alone. If it wasn't my death, or the deaths of those closest to me that preoccupied the minds of the two support groups, I would not be resentful.

This morning someone dumped my glass of water sitting on the counter. My ddI was dissolving in it. Takes a half-hour. Fuck it. Today I go without drugs. I'm concentrating to bring myself down from the highest level of rage I have felt yet on this trip.

[11/17/92 New York. Morning, 11:10 A.M.]

Must document the last days of the trip before returning to work.

On Sunday, 11/15, we woke up to find that the ship's batteries were not charging. This made everyone tense, Peter most of all. The captain's mood guides the crew. Decided to sail to Peter Island where we could charge the batteries on shore power for a few hours while we did mushrooms on the beach.

We moored at the dock, went ashore. Peter went off on his own to read newspapers in the hotel lobby. Frustrated, the rest of us walked to the beach. Peter did not follow and, after what seemed like an hour, feeling guilty, some of us went to find him. Mark and I stayed with the stuff and went swimming. The others rescued Peter from being alone at the peak of his mushroom trip. He was angry. Felt abandoned. No doubt this will be an issue the group addresses later. We all tripped except for Spencer, who went off to have sex with a sailor in the public bathroom of the beach bar. The mushroom trip was amazing. I felt guilty, but the pleasure reigned over the insurgent forces of the superego. The shrooms were strong, came on fast. Laughed hysterically at whatever struck me as funny—including almost everything. High, I realized that all my anxieties are shallow preoccupations that draw my mind away from my one primary concern, my mortality. Earlier, stoned on pot, I steered the boat, sailing toward the horizon. I repeated to myself the same sentence several times, "I am the captain of my ship." The moment was predestined. All the recent moments of my life, the past five years, added up to this one. So it seemed.

I navigated the drug trip better than ever before. I took care of myself. Wouldn't let my mind focus on memories of sad events. Purposely did not stare at my skin. Never look at your own skin on mushrooms. It takes on a translucency much like wax medical models. You become the visible man. Pores open up to reveal veins coursing with blood. You are mere flesh threatened with decay. Better to stare at trees or the water. Clouds. Perhaps sobriety and abstinence are not the same thing. I can take care of myself now. I used to get out of control. Drugs gave me an excuse to force others to take care of me. I couldn't do that to the members of my group. I couldn't let myself fall into a pathetic state, demanding that they care for me. But now I return to New York, feeling anxious, wasted, and afraid to get back to my life. Guilty about the drugs. No. Afraid to admit that I did the drugs without regret. Broke out with blisters on my face from the sun. I look tired and plump. Too much junk food on this trip.

On the last night after dinner we gathered on one side of the boat. All the lights on deck were directed at one point in the dark water. Spencer tore bits of chicken off a carcass and threw them into the lit section of water. A spotlight awaiting the arrival of a special guest. Everyone leaned over the side railing looking for signs of sea life. We were summoning sharks. The guide book reported that sand sharks swim these waters and night is their feeding time. We made jokes all week about not swimming at night for fear of *JAWS.* It came. A small sand shark, four to five feet in length. We squealed. It remained with us as long as our leftovers continued to litter the water. We were ecstatic at proving a fact we were certain of—sharks do swim those waters. We all knew what lay beneath the surface. So easily we drew it out.

On the last day, Monday, everyone was grouchy. Fist fights almost broke out. Peter scheduled a six-hour lay-over in San Juan. Said it couldn't be any other way, but he seemed very happy for the opportunity to gamble at a casino. We split into two groups at the airport: three who wanted, or were resigned, to stay in San Juan until our evening flight and three who would try to get an earlier flight. Mark had the most urgent reason for going back earlier. The next morning, he had to speak in Washington at a conference concerning AIDS drug research. On his birthday. No flights were available. Some of us could not look others in the face. A murder seemed possible. We all went to a hotel near the airport. Some ate and drank by the pool while others gambled. Peter taught me how to shoot craps. I rolled the dice for him, winning at first and then wiping him out. I lost forty dollars of my own money.

In Newark waiting for our bags, Peter said he was disappointed that we would all never be anything more than a support group. He had hoped we would all develop deep friendships. I told him that we had: it takes time and work. David was right. On this trip, we learned how to play together.

On Monday morning, before we sailed the boat to the last dock of the trip, I shot my best video. I was hanging out of the speeding dinghy, balancing the steady-cam, flying around the boat. I took sweeping shots of the *Tucket Mist.*

Dense Moments

6

Originally published as "Dense Moments," in *Uncontrollable Bodies*, eds. Rodney Sappington and Tyler Stawlings (Seattle: Bay Press, 1994), pp. 25–43.

I DON'T WRITE SCREENPLAYS, PER SE. *I write literary pieces that I adapt for the screen. This text served as the guide for my movie* Fast Trip, Long Drop. *Much of it appears in the movie as a series of monologues. The original title for the project, both the text and the movie, was "Dense Moments without Reason." The movie that I eventually made borrowed its title from a newspaper headline. The first paragraph was inspired by the opening lines of Dostoyevsky's* Notes from Underground.

Chapter 6

Dense Moments

I'm sick and I don't want a cure. I like my illness. It's just as much a part of me as any of my other characteristics. I identify as my illness. Today, I feel relatively fine. Probably won't see thirty. Living with infection, me and millions of other people worldwide. I have a disease, an infection that horrifies the uninfected for two reasons. First, there is no cure. Second, the routes of transmission are well known. Sex. Intravenous drugs. Pregnancy, mother to child. Pleasurable, life-affirming things. The kinds of things people have guilt about regardless of their association with this disease. The knowledge of my infection coupled with the careful monitoring of the state of my immune system forces me to face a simple fact: I will die. Of course, I may not. Like everyone else, I could get hit by a car, be murdered, kill myself. Barring these contingencies, it is almost certain that I will die of this disease. I don't know when. Perhaps there will be a cure. Perhaps I can successfully fight the infections my failing immune system will be increasingly unable to fight. More contingencies. Fact is, I don't know when, but I'll die of it.

I've lived these twenty-eight years motivated by a strong desire to change the world, occasionally disrupted by bouts of indolence. This is one of those periods marked by hopelessness. The only activity I can perform without disgust is storytelling. That makes me kind of religious. I don't believe in god, but I have great faith in the power of testimony. Not confession. There are differences, very significant to me, between the confession and the testimony. Through testimony one bears witness to one's own experiences to one's self. Through confession one relinquishes responsibility for bearing witness to and for one's self with the hope that some force greater than one's self will bear away the responsibilities for one's actions. The testimony is the story of a survivor. The confession is the story of a sinner. Both are motivated by guilt. If the survivor does not bear witness to his experience, he may blame himself for the pain he feels despite the fact that the pain was caused by another person's actions. If the sinner does not reveal the nature of his sins, he will suffer the consequences of his actions through punishment inflicted by god. The testimony is secular. The confession is religious. Each can involve the other. The testimony is offered to an other, who listens. The confession is posed to an other who has the power to punish or forgive. They are two distinctly different acts because the precondition for the testimony is a historical cause and the precondition for the confession is a subjective cause. Psychoanalysis engenders both confession and testimony by making subjectivity historical and history subjective. Confession presupposes guilt. Testimony presupposes innocence. Coming out is a form of testimony. Recovery is a form of testimony. Disclosing one's HIV status is a form of testimony. All of these can take the form of confession. Testimony is a means of gaining sovereignty of the self. Confession subjugates the self to a sovereign force. A testimony that leads to confession recapitulates repression. A testimony, performed successfully, can lead toward liberation. (An idealization.) A testimony once started cannot cease. The telling must continue. A confession implies an end, but it is an endless repetition. I want to assume the largest measure of responsibility for myself possible. This can be earned only through a greater understanding of my limits: the limits of my thinking, my actions, my expressions. This is a testimony.

For an entire year I woke up at precisely 9:20 A.M.—the exact time Ray died—without fail. I watched Ray die. One night I went by the hospital to see him. He hadn't recognized anyone for about two weeks. When I came into the room, I knew he was going to die that night. I kept saying to his mother that I would leave, but I remained. I wanted to see him die. Shit. I'd given so much energy and time to his survival, he owed me this. I'd never seen anyone die and this was my opportunity. Later, I realized that I had to witness his death. I wouldn't believe it if I wasn't there. I'd watched Ray give up life at an infinitesimal pace. If I didn't see this to the end I'd feel an inconclusiveness, a suspension of belief, an absence, not a loss—forever. When he was gone, his lack of presence was total. I said to myself, There's nothing. There's nothing. I kissed the forehead that for months had been oily with sweat. It was cool and dry. I didn't make the connection between the exact time of my witnessing Ray's death and the particularity of my sleep disorder until I woke up on November 9, 1991, at 9:20 in the morning, the one-year anniversary of Ray's death. I haven't woken up from sleep at that time of day since. Watching Ray's death corrupted my innocence. Ended my unquestioning faith that every next breath will come.

I spent all night watching him die. Every few minutes asking the nurse to increase the morphine drip. A few days earlier, the decision had been made to take him off all medication except pain killers. At some point in the early morning, the nurse had increased the morphine to the legal limit. When asked to continue, he looked at us angrily and said, "This is pain control, not euthanasia!" and abruptly walked out. I thought that I'd get up off the fucking chair and just increase the dose myself. I'd seen the nurse do it often enough. The liquid dripped through the tube attached to Ray's arm like sand through an hourglass. Die. Just die. He'd been alive but gone for an immeasurable period of time. I'd sit bedside watching, waiting for him to make some noise, some articulation, a string of sounds I could recognize as Ray's speech, not satisfied for days and now I wanted done with it.

Ray gave me a present two weeks before he died. He asked his sister to buy me a copy of Artaud's *To Have Done with the Judgment of God*. He requested that she inscribe the inside cover of the book: *Dear Gregg, To our future shared transgressions. Love always, Ray.* He had an enormous ego. Its size was completely justified by the immensity of his brilliance. Our friendship was based on our arguments. We loved to best each other by quoting theory to support our own frail positions. Ray was California—a handsome Chicano fag with brown skin, long black hair, beard, pronounced cheekbones. He posed in costume as Christ on more than one occasion with great realness.

I must remind myself constantly that murderous feelings toward the sick and dying are common. When he died I wailed. Stuff came up I didn't

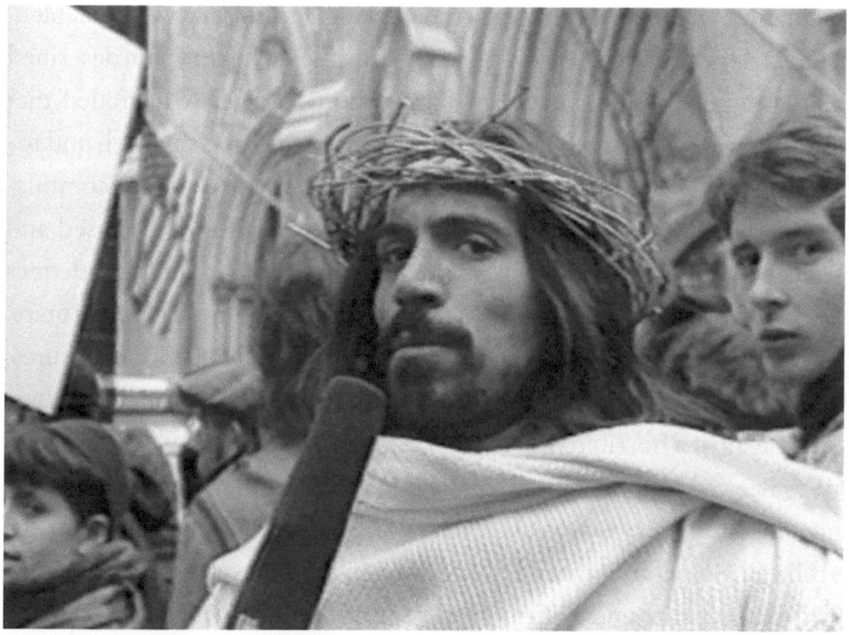

Figure 6.1 Ray Navarro. From *Like a Prayer,* DIVA TV, 1989.

think I contained. And relief. I finally had permission to grieve. Standing over Ray's barely living dying body, I wouldn't allow myself to acknowledge his coming death. It felt like betrayal. Aware that he would die, hopeless, I remained a present witness to his survival until the end.

Do you believe in the possibility of witness? Is it still possible to bear witness to another person's struggle? In *Survival in Auschwitz,* Primo Levi called the camps a laboratory. He described them as an arena of experimentation where modern forms of suffering and misery were patented. The Nazis produced a new type of alienation. Levi, the survivor, described a situation so miserable, in which living conditions were so degraded, that it was impossible to turn to another person in the same situation and together acknowledge the level of misery. The oppression was total, commiseration was impossible. The possibilities of witness were foreclosed and some people drowned, lost in a vast abyss, alone. This situation defines fascism for me. This is hell. This is not my reality; it's my worst nightmare. Those hardest hit by AIDS have struggled to prevent such foreclosures. We've organized ourselves into groups and institutions, formed communities against a horrible violence.

Been in a support group of the infected for over a year. Six white gay men meeting every two weeks, each taking his turn talking while the others listen. Sometimes when I'm speaking in my support group, the familiarity, the repetitiveness, of my monologue frustrates me. The others in the group have heard it all before. I'm fairly articulate about my situation: I'm lonely. Very lonely. Safer sex can be good once you get the hang of it. Intimacy, that's where the real trouble is. Who wants a lover who could die? Who wants a lover who is constantly being reminded of his mortality? I don't trust people who want to be in a relationship with me. I don't get it. Why would they? I don't want to fall in love with someone infected, sick, whatever. I guess it's not a matter of choice. You fall in love with whomever you fall in love with. Of course, I could always run. Bolt. Head for the hills. I have in the past. Being HIV-positive, I'm not supposed to feel this way, right? The correct position: People with HIV/AIDS are capable of everything healthy people are—sex, love. Well, that's a nice bit of denial. I'm not living a normal life, am I? Does everyone think about their death all the time? Consciously? A friend, HIV-negative, straight, told me, "Look, everyone's gonna die. I could go out in the street and get hit by a bus." "I wish you would," was the first thought to come to mind. I didn't say it. She was just trying to be a friend. Probably saying it for her benefit more than mine. Why can't I fight for myself? I hear other people with HIV complain about the HIV-negative world. "They won't have sex with us." "They won't love us." Some positives limit all their sexual and amorous relations to other positives. Is that possible? Isn't that like arbitrarily limiting your desire to only people with hazel eyes? I could understand that, actually.

Representing ourselves, to each other, we defy the representational limits we are forced to adopt. The ways they imagine us on TV have changed over the years. At first, in the early eighties, we were presented as darkly lit or scrambled faces, sometimes sitting behind potted palms. Pictured as criminals, terrorists, and prostitutes. In the mid-eighties, we began to appear without disguises seated next to talk show hosts. We were allowed to speak of our experiences, but only to the host, like we were reporting on some faraway event, another culture. We were still a phenomenon to be observed by a general public. Of course, this setup functioned to reaffirm the boundaries between us and the general public, to assure the audience that there was no threat to them. We haven't seen a person with the disease looking out beyond the TV screen into the television audience and addressing other people with it, forcing the realization that there are infected people watching television, part of the audience, part of the public. He's handsome. White. Well-groomed, but casual. Gap clothes. HIV-positive.

Close-up. Talking to you in your living room. I am a criminal, a terrorist, a prostitute. The media makers were right about that. I'm a threat. I was fucking him, not something I do often because I prefer to get fucked. I wanted to infect him. The whole purpose of bringing myself to orgasm was to infect him with the virus. The idea of infecting him excited me as I jerked myself off. I shot my semen, dripping coolly drawn lines down the side of my right tit, not seeking out the far reaches of my partner's insides as I had wanted and imagined moments before.

How would you feel if I was your lover? What questions would you have for me? The other is presumed to pose an impossible demand on the subject, who never knows what it is the other wants. What will satisfy the other? People with AIDS and HIV are often pictured as a burden on society imposing impossible demands—on the health care system, the infrastructure, the moral order, the family. How would you feel if I was your lover?

It was the first time I asked a guy to fuck me. 1985. I wanted it bad and I was very scared. We were both very drunk. His cock was immense. I thought it would tear me apart and I wanted that. "Fuck me," I demanded, "just fuck me." He was having trouble getting it up because of the liquor. I got mad. "Fuck me! Can't you fuck me?" I was lying on my stomach in a delirious, semiconscious state. He crammed his half-hard cock into my tense hole. I was near dead drunk, but not relaxed. I was in pain as I felt his cock, finally filled with a credible amount of blood, slowly take up space, filling my ass. He went in and out, progressively going deeper as I tried to mentally stretch my shrinking anus. He suddenly stopped, quietly gasped the word "shit" as I felt his cock going limp. I don't know if he came or not. In the morning, it occurred to me that he should have worn a condom. He died a few years later and I have often thought that this was the instance of my infection. I don't know, he wasn't the last, nor certainly the first, to have my ass. He was just the first person I begged to fuck me. That's something.

I wanted him to fuck me without a condom. I received his cum as a gift. I wished for a legacy that I could receive in the form of a gift—the love and approval of a father. I wanted to achieve his stature. His greatness could be passed to me through his semen. A condom would thwart this transference. Was this the instance of my infection? The trauma always happens after the fact. We know it happened, because of its effects. I know I was infected, because a test shows that I have antibodies to the virus. More tests show that my immune system is compromised. I take experimental medications that produce side effects. All of this adds up to the fact of my infection, an event I can never locate in time with any certainty. It's like the time my father left us. This is a primary event in my life, an event that is interpreted and made more significant by events that happened to me later. In many ways, all the significant events in my life confer new meaning on the primary event: the loss of my father.

I was twenty-three years old when I thought I had found what I'd been looking for all my life—a feeling of belonging. I joined the AIDS Coalition To Unleash Power, a diverse nonpartisan group united in anger and committed to direct action to end the AIDS crisis. A cause. What brought me to this group was my increasing awareness of the epidemic and its implications for my future. Guilty and scared, I knew that the sex I was having, particularly anal-receptive sex, had possibly exposed me to a newly identified virus. That the meetings of the activist group were held at the Lesbian and Gay Community Center taught me something. The gay community was the only place to go to get information about this disease. More than just information—support. I had never wanted a sexual identity. I liked sex with men and women and I was successful at both. The possibility of exposure, my concerns and fears about it, centered around the fact that I enjoyed and often practiced what was listed as the most high-risk activity. A homosexual act. I don't know when exactly, but sometime shortly after entering the community center I decided that I had better become a part of this community if I was going to get the information and support I needed to think about this illness.

I tested positive on the same day an ACT UP meeting was scheduled. That night I had to speak at the meeting about a demonstration I had been organizing. It was a protest at City Hall concerning the lack of availability of drug-addiction treatment and the lack of a clean needle exchange program in New York City. I decided that I would admit publicly at the meeting that I had just tested HIV-positive. I was so pissed off that I had to deal with this awful shit that I was going to make everyone deal with it. I wasn't going to own this alone. It would be easier to tell everyone this way. Then I wouldn't have to face any one person to tell him or her the news. Turn the public into the private.

The room was packed with about four hundred people. I stood nervously rocking back and forth on my heels, staring directly down into my notes scribbled on a yellow pad. I started slowly in a low quivering voice: "Next week, on Tuesday, we are going to have a demonstration that addresses issues we as a group have not addressed before. We are going to deal with AIDS and substance abuse. A lot of people have said that this is not an issue for our group . . . and uh . . . a lot of people think this isn't an issue for us . . . and um, uh . . . I just tested HIV-antibody-positive."

There was silence in the room. I heard a couple of gasps.

"I got infected because I have a drinking and drug problem that has prevented me from being able to negotiate and insist on having safe sex. I'm not telling you this to talk about myself. I'm telling you this because I think a lot of other people in this room have had the same experience. Issues of drug use and AIDS are our issues. The connection between drug abuse and safe sex must not be left out of any discussion about AIDS and substance abuse. It's important to recognize this connection because too often the issues are reduced to a single issue of needle use. This reduction legitimates misconceptions about drug use and users. It reinforces the view that IV drug users are alien and criminal. Substance abuse is not an issue of criminal law. The focus should be on treatment and services.

“We’ve got to ask ourselves who are the gays and who are the drug users? Who are the fags and who are the junkies? We have got to seriously question the names and categories used to separate the groups of people hardest hit by this epidemic. We have to take responsibility for these issues. We’re demanding a clean needle exchange program to help IV drug users remain uninfected by HIV until they can get clean. We’re demanding free drug-addiction treatment upon demand to anyone who wants it. So be there next Tuesday at noon.”

I ended with my voice strong, but my hands were shaking. There was silence and then scattered applause. Some people came up to me afterward and thanked me. A couple of people approached me and confided that they, too, had had trouble practicing safe sex when they were drunk. It was a fairly cogent speech, considering the events of the day. I thought I was facing the news head-on. Doing the only thing I could do. Act. I was running. What I did was crazy. Created a storm around me so I wouldn’t have to be emotionally responsible to anyone. Sure, everyone I’d had sex with, whose name I could remember, would find out they’d had sex with someone now infected. Either I’d tell them or, more than likely, they’d hear by word of mouth. I’d taken care of that. But I couldn’t, wouldn’t, deal with the fallout, the real possibility that I had unknowingly infected people. They might be mad at me. Even if I didn’t do it purposefully, they still might be mad. Their anger would be justifiable, I didn’t want to take responsibility for their anger, I didn’t know that I didn’t have to. Just because someone’s angry at you doesn’t necessarily mean that you’re guilty.

But wasn't I? I'd broken up my parents' marriage. A very powerful four-year-old, I was. Capable of mass destruction. I drove my father out of the house. Ruined my mother's life. Seven years old, playing outside with a friend, I point to the man on the porch, my stepfather: "That's not my real dad. My real dad's gone." My mom, sitting next to my stepdad, pulls me by the arm. She is pissed. Tells me never to tell anyone outside the family that he isn't my father. Never. I'd revealed a secret. It was all my fault.

I accept the blame. The guilt I feel greatly affects my actions. After the speech to ACT UP I took on a persona—Gregg Bordowitz, HIV-Antibody-Positive Gay Man. I came out all over the place. Every time I put myself forward as an HIV-Positive Gay Man I was flattening out the terms of my identity to further the cause of an agenda: the enfranchisement of people with HIV and AIDS. I disclosed an aspect of my sexuality, my homosexuality, because it was a factor in my infection. Each time I came out about my HIV status and my sexuality I felt authenticated, legitimated. I felt that my concerns mattered. More than that, my disease and my sexuality, viewed as indistinct by many, became terms with which others identified. Disclosing my status, coming out, I didn't feel alone. I didn't feel sick, perverse. I felt that I was on the side of right and justice. I was enabled to overcome my shame. That's important. A matter of survival. The disclosure would vanquish my guilt temporarily. I had to repeatedly and insistently assert my new identity, fighting against an internal conclusion that my pleasure had led to my death. Through a kind of exhibitionism, I was trying to exorcise the discourse of blame that would judgmentally bring sentence down upon me for getting fucked up the ass, liking it, and getting a fatal disease from it. Where did this discourse exist? Among the homophobes. Among the right wing. And in my own mind. Sometimes, I believe that my homosexuality is a disease and that I deserve to get sick from it. This thought can overtake me at any time. I think it in my dreams. I hear it in the voices of kind friends and see it in the faces of my relatives. It's always present. I am not resigned to it. I fight it. I won't grant it sovereignty. I refuse to be ruled by it. Now, I no longer feel compelled to present myself publicly as HIV-positive. I am not my disease. It's a shallow identity. It doesn't have the history, the significance, of other identities I have, like being gay or Jewish. I was taught as a child that there are two kinds of people in the world—Jews and non-Jews. I thought that my Jewish identity was the aspect of my character that made me different from everyone else. I always felt different, apart, alone. When I was fifteen I realized I was of the "working class." That's what made me different. Went around telling everyone, I'm a socialist. At eighteen, I moved into Manhattan. Lived with my first boyfriend. Realized I was queer. Thought this was what made me different. There was a finality in this realization. I thought that I'd finally figured out why I'd always felt different. Now, I realize that my class identity didn't displace my religious identity, and my sexual identity didn't displace my class identity. I am all these things, and their interrelatedness somehow constitutes my identity. HIV is a disease. That infection has taken on the status of an identity reveals the immense sense of shame we're all operating with in this puritanical culture. Living with HIV is awful. It's terrifying. It's tedious. I don't want to spend the rest of my life being identified as a disease. I am much more than that. Don't reduce me to that. I can no longer reduce myself to that. The shameful feelings behind my status as an infected person still exist, but I no longer need to subordinate my identity to the level of my status to ward off evil, uncertainty, and death. A kind of alchemy, turning shit into gold, stigma into pride.

I often imagine that I am acting in the interests of the public good. I picture this entity as a jury presiding over my pleasure. It's a guilt-ridden fantasy. Who am I acting good for? And who will punish me for evil thoughts? Will Daddy spank me? I hope so. I hope he sticks a big stick up my ass while Mommy watches. Further, she says. Deeper. The conviction with which I act comes from deep-seated rage. I know I have it in me. I have fantasies of murder. As I noted before, I've imagined myself infecting others and I enjoy that fantasy. I don't know what to do with this information. I recognize myself as the subject of these sentences and I'm scared. I'm frightened of death and the fear overtakes my desire.

In a dream, I'm in a Lower East Side apartment lying on a couch in the center of the room. Ray, sick with lesions covering his body, is sitting in the corner, silent. A woman is lying on top of me. We're fucking and just as I'm about to shoot I remember that Ray is in the corner. Then, the woman turns into a man. The dream starts again. We're having sex and just before I climax I see Ray sitting in the corner and the guy on top of me turns into a girl.

I lost my virginity to a girl two years older. She was fast. Gave me a blow job in a duck blind in the woods behind her house on our first date. As she fellated, I tried to reach down her pants to finger her. Told me I didn't have to. This being my first blow job, it never occurred to me that you could get pleasure from someone without giving it back immediately. I felt guilty. Couldn't believe that I was supposed to sit back and enjoy this. Wasn't I the one responsible for the good feelings here?

The times and places of my sexual encounters as a teenager were organized around when and where parents worked. Whose house was empty during the day, at night. Our encounters paralleled the shifts of our parents' jobs. That I had sex with girls and yearned for sex with guys reveals the repressive context of my teenage years; it also reveals the formation of my desires shaped earlier in my life partly by my parents' divorce. I wanted my absent father's love and I depended on my mother's. She depended on my love and approval. I didn't know that then. I grew up thinking it was the duty of every boy to take care of his mother's emotional needs. This duty was a temporary position until my father returned. My stepfather never filled the position. Not through any fault of his own. When my father left he became an entity larger than any human. He became a category.

I would have drunk gasoline and lit my ass on fire if that had been the only way to get out of Long Island. Moved to the city in 1982, the summer I turned eighteen. Started drinking every day. Used to drink with bums on the street. Thought maybe I'd become one. Woke up in a doorway on 34th Street once. Scared me. Tried to go on the wagon. Didn't last long. Managed to keep the habit without going on the street. Don't know how. Wouldn't allow myself to. Learned how to manage the use. First time I did coke was in the YMCA that I lived in with some other art students. School of Visual Arts. Buncha young fags and dykes lying all over each other on a single bed. None of us was self-identified as lesbian or gay. Don't remember much about the actual experience of doing coke for the first time. Moved in with my first boyfriend. First guy to fuck me. When I met him he was wearing a green mod mac with a huge pink triangle sewn onto the back. He had his social security number tattooed onto his forearm like a camp survivor. A punk gesture which greatly contradicted the lyrical color-field paintings he made in the front room of our studio in Cobble Hill, Brooklyn.

Somewhere along the way my values changed. I once held a romantic, devout belief in beauty. I was a painter when I moved to Manhattan. I've always wanted to be an artist. All my life. My paintings were often shown in the cafeteria of P.S. 186. Later, in high school, I spent most of my time in the art rooms making abstract expressionist paintings. I wanted to be Jackson Pollock. When I attended art school I started making monochromatic paintings. Ad Reinhardt. All black. Painting became a task. I realized that I didn't enjoy the act of painting. I loved the act of making meaning. I started painting myself out of my pictures, applying the paint on the canvas with a roller, executing the task as fast as I could. I became more interested in how the object hung on the walls. Then I became fascinated with the walls. First as surface, later as architecture. I went from viewing the gallery as a structure to questioning it as an institution. Who determined what hung on the walls and why? Who attended galleries and why? Whose interests were being served and what did I desire? I began making video because I needed to work in a time-based medium to answer all these questions. The first work was about my sexuality in the context of AIDS. I became interested in AIDS as a political crisis. Protest groups were forming. Videomaking became a means of documenting the emerging movement. Started working collectively to make documentaries. Began writing and publishing critical analyses of my own work. I adopted a set of aesthetic principles to which I was, until recently, committed: reduce the category of beauty to efficacy, the category of form to function, the category of audience to community. Today I'm sitting here writing myself out of the categories I reduced myself to.

I stopped drinking and doing drugs for pleasure, substituting an entirely different pharmacopoeia: Bactrim, AZT, Zovirax, ddC, ddI. I've lived with HIV for four years and I've remained relatively asymptomatic for AIDS. Lots of colds, a few minor skin rashes, warts, but no opportunistic infections. I initially took AZT—an antiviral drug that slows the progress of HIV replication—for over a year, every four hours. I was part of the beeper generation. Carried my AZT in a box with a timer that beeped every four hours to remind me to take the pills. I waited for the beeper to sound

in public places, anticipating the embarrassment it would cause me. Eventually, I stopped using the beeper. Removed the batteries. What the fuck, they don't know if this works, who cares if I take it late, early, whatever.

I take Bactrim to prevent pneumocystis carinii pneumonia. I've added Zovirax to my regimen because theoretically it prevents infections that could threaten my eyesight, or cause severe fatigue. It's also a herpes treatment. At this point I can no longer take AZT because the cumulative effect of its toxicity adversely affected my liver. So, I started to take ddC—an experimental antiviral that I got through my doctor as part of a study to measure the drug's efficacy. Label on the bottle: *Dideoxycytidine has been associated with contact sensitivity. Persons handling this drug should take measures to avoid prolonged contact with tablets or tablet dust.* How do you take a drug you're not supposed to touch? These drugs yield no pleasurable effects. Side effects: AZT: nausea, growling stomach-empty-speediness. ddC: loss of feeling in the feet and hands, signs of neuropathy. I can't take ddC anymore. Dead hands are not compatible with the purchase of a laptop. My hands fell asleep, a long nap. I went off the drug and all the feeling came back.

I feel discouraged but I don't think I'm going to die. It's not because I'm brave. I just can't wrap my mind around death. It's still abstract to me. Like my T-cell counts are on paper but I'm feeling fine. The blood tests I get every three months count the number of T cells I have. They're lymphocytes, the cells that HIV attacks. So, it's important to know your number because if it's a low number you may be in trouble: it means your immune system can't respond. Anyway, my T cells are low on paper but I'm feeling fine, so it's all in the abstract.

I have a range of emotions that goes from anger to rage. I'm proud of my anger. I want to work with it, develop it, make it more powerful. Sometimes, it's all I have. I hate some of the spiritual crap people try to hand me to calm me down—like everything happens for a reason. There's no reason, no reason at all for why I'm HIV-positive, why some people get sick, why some people die. No reason.

In the spring of 1988. March and April. I tested HIV-antibody-positive. Stopped drinking and doing drugs. And I told my parents I am gay. I went out to their house on Long Island to talk to them. They live in what is called a "development"—rows of houses attached to one another within a maze of cul-de-sacs. Strathmore Court. At the time, my stepfather was working any fix-it job he could get and my mother was working as a salesperson in a department store. My sister was in high school. Strange that I would wait to talk to them about my sexuality until after having tested HIV-antibody-positive. I knew that I wasn't going to let them know about my HIV test. First, I would tell them proudly that I was gay. Once they accepted that, if they accepted it, I would, sometime in the near future, talk to them about AIDS. (I didn't tell them about being HIV-infected until over a year later.) I didn't want them to associate my homosexuality with illness. Actually, it was I who didn't want to associate my homosexuality with illness. Fantasies of telling my family about my life on my deathbed had become a preoccupation. I would avoid this scenario regardless of how painful it would be to confront my parents.

The day I came out, I was sitting with my parents at the kitchen table. My sister was upstairs watching TV. My parents must have sensed that I was going to broach some serious topic, because if I weren't I would have been upstairs watching TV too. Throughout my life, members of my family always occupied the same seats at the kitchen table. I sat on the same side as my mother, facing my stepfather. On this day, I occupied the seat my sister usually sat in, facing my mother, my stepfather to my left. I told them. I said that there was something they should know and accept about me if they expected me to include them in my life. I am gay. My mother burst into tears. My stepfather got up to pace. My mother couldn't stop crying for about two hours. My stepfather surprised me with his response. It was OK as far as he was concerned. Attempting to quiet my mother, he appealed to her to look at the bright side: "Linda, Linda, look. Come on, stop crying. Look, he didn't kill anybody, and he's not a drug addict," he said emphatically looking at me for assurance. At least I hadn't killed anybody. At some point my sister came downstairs to see what was happening. Looking at my mother, who was trying to contain her sobs, she asked what was wrong. I looked at her and said that I had just told our parents that I am gay. She started crying, too, like she'd been cued. I thought to myself, the whole thing feels scripted. My sister must have felt implicated. Maybe this meant she was queer. Maybe she thought she'd have to tell people at school. I still don't know; we haven't talked about it since. Over time my parents have come to deal with it. They're now aware that I have this infection, although their response to learning this was much less emotional than my coming out. I thought it should have been more painful. I don't think they realized the implications, and I gave them a very optimistic picture. I didn't admit to them that I fear my own death in the next few years. I lied. Told them it was like diabetes. I can keep it under control. I fed them the bullshit I'd love to hear someone else tell me, and the things I knew they were capable of hearing. I'm tired of representing the situation in ways that take care of the needs of the listener. Fuck you. I know it's not my fault, but I'm angry at you. Testimony. Confession. Why should I have to explain it all to you? I need you. LISTEN TO ME. Don't go. Don't . . . When Ray was dying, he became extremely religious. He hadn't been religious, was even somewhat antireligious, and I found myself in a predicament: I wanted to be supportive because I loved my friend, but I don't believe in god. At his bedside, we would talk about god often. After a long silence, with tears in his eyes, in a child's voice begging permission, he asked me, "Can I believe in god after I've read Nietzsche?" Pause. *God is dead. He remains dead. And we have killed him.* We both had to laugh at the high level of pretension behind that question. We weren't prepared for this. The critical theory we valued so much had failed us. Not because of its inadequacy, because of its limits. We, Ray talking, I listening, had come up against the contingencies we had until then disavowed. And why not?

He was twenty-six then, so was I, and our heads were crowned with the twisted branches of our own ambitious weaving. You can have only a very inadequate knowledge of the duration of other bodies.

I was Bar Mitzvahed in an orthodox temple. It was the cheapest. My grandfather wanted to pay, therefore he sent me to an orthodox temple. The musty smell of old books and the company of men. It was a formative experience. I was such a good student that for my Bar Mitzvah I performed, in addition to my haftorah, the entire Shabbat service. I professed a deeply felt belief in god that suffered and failed many tests after my Bar Mitzvah. Still, the entire framework of my thinking presupposes the category of god. Retain the category of god in one's thinking as a category of the unknown, as an arena of forces that lie outside, or on the periphery of comprehension. Something more than mere random variables and chance. Forces motivated without intention. No will. Forces not motivated by a human mind, but motivated, nonetheless. Arbitrary and motivated. God is a structural necessity. Spinoza: *God is the immanent, not the transitive, cause of things.* God has neither intention nor will. The category of god can be retained, but its human image must vanish. It's a category of mystery composed of forces beyond understanding. Amoral. Nonjudgmental. Causal. Can one pray to it? No. What can one do? Resign to it. There are some things beyond our control, beyond our understanding.

In the spring of 1988. March and April. I tested positive. Stopped drinking and doing drugs. And I told my parents I am gay. This was the densest moment of my life. The moment when I first realized that what matters is the meaning I make of my life. The moment when I began to write my own story. Yes, I am the subject of these sentences. My story began and now it ends with a single explanatory event in mind. The death of my father. It is for his eyes this is written. For his ears this is told. His imagined interest. That it can only be imagined causes me great pain. Probably always will. I can live with that pain. I don't have to suffer for it. Before the spring of 1988, I was very far away from believing this.

I was eight or nine when my mother tried to run away with my stepfather's best friend. One morning I was awakened by the sounds of yelling and shuffling coming from the kitchen in our Queens apartment. I walked into the kitchen to see my stepfather in his pajamas holding a steak knife to his chest and crying, "Take it out. Go ahead, take my heart, too. Go ahead." My mom was shrieking for him to put the knife down. John, my stepfather's best friend, was standing there. He said something too, like, "Be cool man. Be cool." All three of them stopped dead looking at me. I'm not clear on what happened next. I remember holding on to my stepfather and wailing, "I don't want to go." I didn't want to lose him. We left with suitcases and some of my toys. G.I. Joe. My sister was just an infant then. That night at John's house I asked my mom if this was going to happen again, implying that this father-changing thing was becoming a routine. She laughed and started to cry. Don't remember how long we stayed with John. Driving in the car, John asked me if I was angry. He told me it was OK if I was mad at him, it was OK even if I was mad at my mom. I mumbled that I was OK. One night my stepfather showed up with my grandfather and my uncle. The men. After a long talk among everyone concerned—my mom, John, and the men—I was packed up along with my sister into my grandfather's blue Granada. We returned to Queens. I never saw John again. For months, my mother and stepfather held closed-door conversations. For months, maybe years, I misrecognized every strange man who walked down the block toward our building for John. I thought he was coming back to take us away. I had mixed feelings about that. I feared it and I longed for it.

I expected either one of my parents to leave at any moment. I was torn between a strong desire for the love of my father and the love of my mother. I conceived of them as mutually exclusive categories and I tried to demonstrate my love for each without allowing the other to see my efforts. I've spent my adult life bouncing back and forth between relationships with women and relationships with men. Caught between the love of a man and the love of a woman. I've been in that situation many times. Not until very recently have I recognized the logic behind this pattern. These instances exemplify the ways I've developed for coping with the possibilities of loss. If I am torn between two love objects, I always have somewhere to go, and if one decides to withdraw his or her love, I will always have the other. My efforts are calculated to prevent the pain of loss. I expect it like I anticipated my father's death.

Dad, I'm glad you're dead. You're more interesting that way. The only photos I have of my father are a publicity shot when he was twenty, toothful smile, strumming a guitar, and Bar Mitzvah pictures of thirteen-year-old Les wearing tallis. I spent my childhood waiting for my father to return and set things right. I mistook every strange man walking toward me on the street for my father. The Jew lives in an anticipatory present. Always waiting for the Messiah. I've been waiting for my father to return ever since he left. He's dead. And I'm an adult now. I've struggled all my life to be able to write this. It's absurd. So simple. He's not coming back.

My father died when he was thirty. I just turned twenty-nine. All my life I've thought that I am inescapably like my father. In many ways I've acted as I have imagined him to be. I was given a folder of material concerning my father from my paternal grandfather. It contains hundreds of pieces of paper. Newspaper ads for a guitar school he owned. Invitations to recitals. Some pictures. Canceled checks. The accident report concerning my father's death and a photostat of a newspaper account of the accident that killed my father.

Due to a misprint in the *Times News*, Idaho's Largest Evening Newspaper, Twin Falls, Idaho, Monday, September 9, 1974, two paragraphs of an article concerning my father's death were misplaced inside the lead article, concerning Evel Knievel's unsuccessful stunt. The headline of the lead story read:

> FAST TRIP, LONG DROP
> Evel Knievel tried—but failed—to conquer the Snake River Canyon with his steam rocket in the dust and wind late Sunday afternoon.
>
> But, Knievel said later, "to lose a beautiful canyon and river is not to me a real loss."
>
> The rocket fired at 3:44 P.M., about 20 minutes later than scheduled, in front of a jump-site crowd estimated at one-fifth the size expected—about 10,000 people. Perhaps another 10,000 watched from Shoshone Falls, along the rim and from rooftops. . . .
>
> A California man, walking from Shoshone Falls along Falls Avenue late Saturday night, was struck and killed in a car-pedestrian accident. Sheriff's officers said Leslie Hugh Harstein, 30, North Hollywood, a producer of special shows, was killed as he and his wife were walking toward their automobile, which had been left on Desert View Drive.
>
> Hospital officials said Mr. Harsten was apparently killed instantly about 10 p.m. Saturday. Cloyce Edwards, county coroner, said the man died of head injuries and was dead at the scene. He was struck by a pickup truck and camper also traveling west.
>
> . . . Knievel's wife, his three children and numerous relatives watched the launch from the canyon rim. Linda remained silent, according to an observer, during the takeoff, as relatives shouted, "Oh, my god." When the skycycle disappeared behind the rocks, she ran to the edge crying, "Where is it?"
>
> Informed by a reporter her husband was alive, "she just grinned," the reporter said.

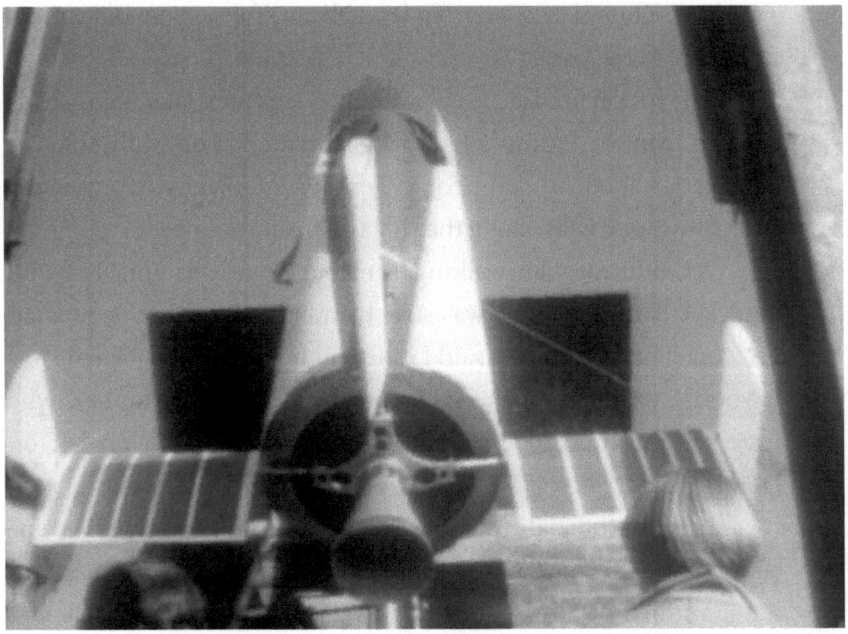

Figure 6.2 Gregg Bordowitz, *Fast Trip, Long Drop*, 1993.

Another strange coincidence—Knievel's wife is named Linda, my mother's name, my father's first wife. I'm his only kid.

> SOME FANS FELT CHEATED
> Sunday night a near riot erupted after a group of campers at the jump site, believed to be unhappy over the failure of Evel Knievel to provide free beer, began burning and tearing up concession stands, fences and automobiles.

A disappointed fan, I am my father's absence. Can we be the subjects of the following sentence? I am the author of this story. Now the author faces his own death. He says, I am the beginning of something, the end of another. A vehicle. A failed rocket. There's a void to be leapt. An impossible void. How can I make it? He's gone. Am I here? The author of this story is already dead. I will tell his story. I am a witness. I will make it my own. Telling it, I survive. Concluding, I will die. Deliverance?

I make plans for my inevitable illness. After Ray died, I moved into an apartment building with an elevator. Ray lived in a walk-up five flights up. I carried him up and down the stairs when it became impossible for him to make the trip. I don't want anyone to have to carry me and I will not be trapped in my apartment on a sunny day for fear of asking friends to carry me out. Some say my pragmatic approach is morbid, but I'm proud of it. I feel like I'm taking care of myself by preparing for the worst. Ray wasn't tested for HIV until he became ill. He found out after the TB when he had about eighty T cells. I was tested well in advance of illness. I'm relatively healthy at the moment but I live with constant anxiety and an acute awareness of my mortality. I think about my funeral sometimes. I like to think that people will miss me. They'll say, "He was brilliant," or, "He was fucked up, but I loved him anyway."

I don't want to die. I've come head up against the actual limiting dimensions of my body. I now realize that though my actions once seemed to extend far out along chains of causality, they never actually got any farther than the surface of my skin. I am scared to die. I am living with this infection. I live in spite of it. I fuck. I love. I'm loved. Eat. Sleep. Shit. Laugh. Living is so much more than biological function; life can be nothing less. I have a life. It's hard-won. But sometimes, I'm miserable and ashamed, deeply ashamed. Have I fit all of this within the frame of the picture? Did all of this come to rest within a single composition? I can feel some force inside me struggling to reach a degree zero. I don't know what constitutes that level of knowledge. I can't tell whether it is a yearning for something, or an urge to cover something up. I'll never reach it. The zero. I can't be nothing. I have a past. I have substance. To nullify it would be suicide, and that is not my intention. I want to live unfettered by the enormous weight of my substantiality. To sublate. Abandon the old self—the one with the quirky ways that are no longer sufficient in and of themselves to answer life's quirks. Nine fucking twenty A.M. and I have to change. I'm too many things. Too many contradictions. Too many people. I'm writing and I'm reading. I'm gay and I'm straight. Working-class and bourgeois. Jewish and American. Faithful and hopeless. Ethical and evil. Reasonable and irrational. Testifying and confessing. Living and dying. Unresolved, irreconcilable, inconclusive. Contingent. Mortal. Ambivalent. And not resigned.

Present Tense

7

Originally published as "Present Tense," in *Processed Lives: Gender and Technology in Everyday Life,* eds. Jennifer Terry and Melody Calvert (London and New York: Routledge, 1997), pp. 104–105. Minor revisions have been made for consistency.

I WANTED TO EXPLORE THE ASSOCIATIONS *set into motion by a medical procedure, necessitated by chronic diarrhea, diagnosed as lymphadnopathy in the intestinal tract. I was heavily sedated, but awake, throughout the medical procedure. The space of the operating room took on the many-layered topography of the psyche. After the exploratory procedure the doctor came into the recovery room with pictures of my intestines. The entire operation was recorded on video. I declined to take the pictures and prevented myself from asking for the video. I knew that if I did, I'd use them, and I didn't want to. I never wanted to reduce the exploratory nature of my work to such a literal exposition. I preferred a textual description that wouldn't be overwhelmed by a sensational depiction of my body's interior—that can be encountered only as an abstraction through language and never a truth reduced to biological documentation.*

Chapter 7

Present Tense

The colonoscopy is more a day trip than a journey into night. First of all, I'm awake and I can watch on the monitors the probe's progress into an alternating white and pink zone, tissue and substance, seemingly dry, although liquid runs out of my ass like a birth upon the insertion of the tube. Me and the doctor are now asshole buddies. Three female nurses witness the intimate act. I think, I can take this, I've had larger. The Demerol does the job, making me the dumb one among the skilled technicians. All I have to do is lie still. I am the reason for this congregation. I am vulnerable. I am in control. The feelings contradict themselves as I lay open. I say *I'm in pain, I need more stuff,* like a rat hitting the feeder bar for more relief and like a king calling for more libations. I am a victim, I am a lord. The proximity of death, either a fantasy or an actual situation makes one feel both supreme and supremely humble. David accompanies me to the hospital. He watches me walk out of the waiting room into the dressing room. I return dressed in the hospital gown, humiliated. Later, he says to me, *you arrive a person and they turn you into a patient.* He is waiting for me in the recovery room. I am still very high. He gets me apple juice. We wait for the doctor for two hours. The doctor arrives with polaroids of my intestine. He says, *I'd say that's the wildest case of lymphadnopathy I'd ever seen 'cept I've seen so many.*

I want to write like a poet about my asshole. I want to attribute to it the clinch of a jaw, the sharpness of teeth, a mind of its own. I can't. It burns. My asshole burns from the acids of my stomach. The intestinal system responds to the stimulation of the swollen nodes surrounding it. In an effort to relieve itself of the irritation and the increased amount of lymph in the area, I shit. The asshole is a conduit for diarrhea, that's all. It burns constantly, reminding me it exists. If anything, I pity the organ. The asshole, the intestine, just doing their jobs, fooled into action by a trickster virus that makes the body function in good faith against itself. Pure evil. Without intention. One life-form perverts the other for its own ends . . . survival.

The actual conditions of illness make me a failure as a poet for I can see no beauty in this decay. I can see no meaning in it. This is simply happening. It happens to me. That sentence seems odd; it is difficult for me to imagine myself the subject of that sentence. The I that is writing now does not understand itself to be the me of that sentence. I am the witness to my body's history. I watch as it becomes ill, from some safe distance, like watching the news on television. I'm lying on my side with a long thin probe three feet snaked into my intestines and I'm watching it all on TV. The doctor's head is turned to watch the monitor as he pushes the wire further into me. The nurses stare at the screen. For a moment, I'm ten years old, sitting in the living room, watching television with my mom, my step-dad and my sister. I'm in a lot of pain. I'm an angry kid. I've got a lot going on inside me and I feel like everyone is turned away from me, ignoring me, watching TV. I've seen exploratory images of the insides of bodies on TV medical programs. I am prepared for this new knowledge. Television prepares us. We are well prepared. The colon on the screen could be any colon. If I weren't lying here, heavily sedated, a burning sensation in my gut and all these witnesses, you couldn't convince me of the fact that the image on the screen refers to me. All this evidence proves nothing. I am well. I am in control. I am the I that determines what I am and what I am not. I am not the image of my intestine. I am not an asshole, but the image of a live rotting corpse—devoid of waste but for the wasting.

I do not have language at my disposal. It disposes of me. I want to give myself up to it. To be present in every word I say and to say everything I can now. A crime is committed and no one speaks to stop it. Something feels wrong. We face a daily violence. I wash, I get pimples. I use soap, I get pimples. I get pimples. Get strong. Get gentle. Rediscover the wonder. You have to be picky these days. You can't trust everybody.

8

New York Was Yesterday

THE FOLLOWING TEXTS WERE SELECTED *from an ongoing column written for the journal* Documents *between 1996–2000. The column was completed a year before the tragedy of September 11. Had I continued writing it during that disaster, the notion of New York's passing would have become anathema to me.*

The title for my column was adapted from Janet Flanner's letters to The New Yorker *magazine, written between 1925 and 1939, and collected under the title* Paris Was Yesterday. *Flanner's Paris was a waning center of creative fomentation very different from Walter Benjamin's "Paris, Capital of the Nineteenth Century," another source I kept in mind.*

In the middle of writing this series, I moved to Chicago for love and employment. My literary sense of loss was supplanted by an actual period of mourning for the city I'd lived in all my life, until I was thirty-five.

Chapter 8

New York Was Yesterday

[Lonely Is the City]

To get a view of Manhattan you have to leave. My girlfriend Claire lives under the Brooklyn Bridge on the Brooklyn side. An enviable location. Sometimes, when I leave her building in the morning I follow the line of the bridge to the skyline on the other side of the river—a view that epitomizes

Figure 8.1 Zoe Leonard, "Shmura Matzoh Bakery." © Zoe Leonard, from an ongoing series begun in 1998.

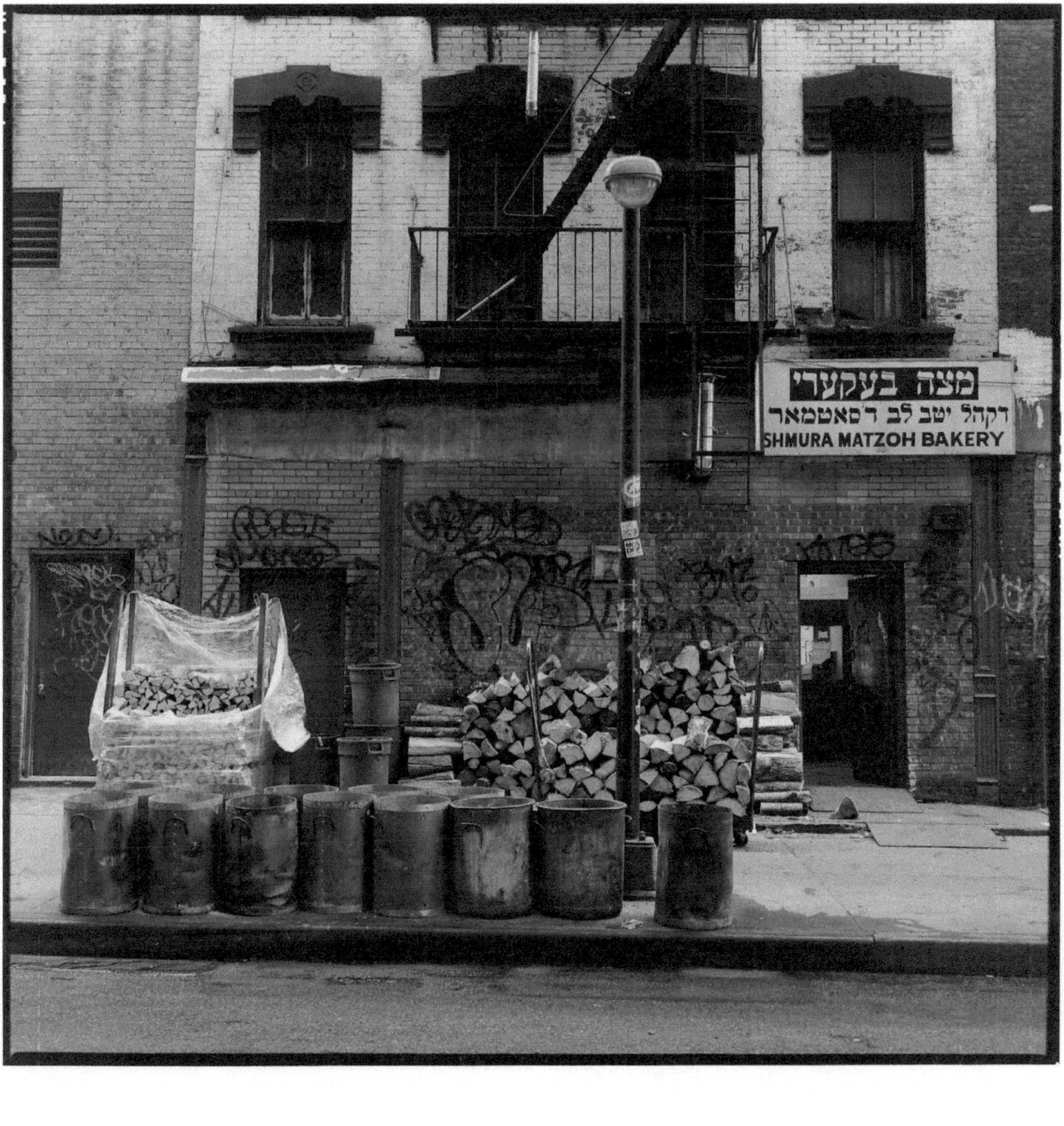
מצה בעקערי
דקהל יטב לב ד׳סאטמאר
SHMURA MATZOH BAKERY

the yearning a borough kid feels when he knows his future is to be made there. I came to Manhattan to be an artist, like Pollock, like Warhol. Blame Emile de Antonio. *Painters Painting* was an effective recruiting film. I, like all of my peers, came here with an established set of models in place. A set of histories already documented. And we managed to make some of our own history—the East Village, ACT UP . . . Some of us are arrested by our nostalgia for only a few short years ago.

Today, the sky is a steel gray wash. The sun, a spot weld intolerably bright. I crawl along the day's agenda, oppressed by the amount of time it takes to get from here to there. One task leads to the next. Wandering exhausts me—today I am the composition of a gas. Weightless between turnstiles, seeping, floating above the concrete, mingling with fumes and odors made fresh by the newly arrived season. The motion of bodies passing around me shapes me, contains me. I must resist the urge to disperse. The street walls are a comfort. They block vistas, making it easy to keep the eyes focused in one direction. The flat facades separated by thin lines between mortar and stone. Brick meets granite meets marble. At the corner, a shaft of light, a slice of sky, like a door cracked open for a moment.

Think of *Vir Heroicus Sublimis,* by Barnett Newman, one of the most beautiful paintings in the collection of the Museum of Modern Art. I am convinced that it could not have been painted anywhere except New York City. The attention to line, monumental scale, the emphasis on surface, are idioms derived from an urban landscape. The painters of the New York School were confronted by a frustrated perspective.

You can get a nice view from the top of the Empire State Building, but that's not the quotidian experience of a New Yorker. Everything great happens on the street. Trolling along, one finds many parcels of space yet to be filled, altered, supplemented. These signs of potential give a citizen a sense of hope. Look closer and cracks appear in the walls. The structures are buckling under the weight of aspiration. One wonders if anything new can survive the surrounding decay. In the natural world new plants thrive off the demise of others.

Visit the Sheep Meadow in Central Park. The city looks like a forest where buildings rise out of the tree tops. It's a wonder how the trunks support the weight of iron and stone—unclear how the construction emerges from the growth. A cellulose much sturdier than marble grows these girders and beams. The skyline isn't an imposition on the plants, it grows out of them. They stem from a common seed. Inhabitants climb the trunks to elevators that carry them to their dwellings. I am at peace with this notion. I accept the idea that our lives are lived out through institutions organic to the soil; relieved to see a vegetative foundation for human accomplishment.

I am at a loss. The first-person singular pronoun shares the same fate as the skyscraper. Rem Koolhaas wrote that the problem of designing a monolithic structure to house a corporate enterprise is an outmoded concern. The architect must conceive of big structures to connect newly forming matrices. He notes that cities expand as travel moves faster. Distances are shortening to include the suburbs within newly drawn urban limits. A new design problem: how to map the overlapping movements of whole populations sharing the same urban space. I'm ambivalent about Koolhaas. He's the only artistic mind working with the forces determining the shape of our future. He reminds me of Orson Welles's character in *The Third Man* looking down on a crowd of people from the top of a Ferris wheel, pondering the significance of one small dot vanishing.

I is a morbid pronouncement at the end of the century. I wish to represent many, in the singular I cannot speak. Will not. As though my silence will convene stadiums. I'll stand before the microphone, wordless. Shrill fuzzy feedback will echo through the silence. The crowd will stir in anticipation of what I might say. A fantasy of countless fans is not enough to produce music from the instrument of an untrained player. Arrogance cannot entertain alone. A familiar face in the crowd humbles. Talent performs for two, or three. The others eavesdrop on the intimate. Sing?! How dare I? A burden on the neighborhood. A car alarm sounds miserable with the presumption of its own necessity. People are indifferent or annoyed by such foolishness. Turn it off. "I" is a syndicated talk show. "We" is a corporate enterprise. Factors in an equation. Pronouns in a sentence. Notations, a couple of keystrokes, commands. Do this. Feel that. American culture is a funeral.

Health has displaced the weather as the most commonly discussed topic. Can't walk a block in Chelsea without comparing notes on the latest protease inhibitors. At dinner we discuss side effects: nausea, fatigue, headaches. Irritability isn't on the list but it should be. Each of us adheres to a different regimen according to the chemical composition of our medicine. I must take my pills one hour before and two hours after a meal. My stomach must be empty. Two 400mg pills three times daily, in addition to the seventeen pills spread throughout the day. Eight glasses of water to keep them all moving through the system. Drinking is not motivated by thirst. Eating is no longer a direct response to hunger. I follow orders. And I am lucky. The simple truth about AIDS: if you can afford treatment you live longer. If you can't, you die.

I'm tired. Maybe that's why there are so many coffee bars. Everyone's given everything else up. Can't smoke, can't drink, might as well stay awake. Might as well sleep. We are fatigued. Our faces are drawn downward by our smiles. We bare our teeth. We have the look of the endangered. The city makes too many demands on us. We feel insufficient to its needs. It takes a toll.

Now a common topic of discussion is when and how to leave. Some have managed to escape. Zoe, a native New Yorker, is living in Alaska for an unspecified period of time. Mark and Morgan keep an exquisite space in Tribeca, but he's off traveling to Europe more than he's here, and Morgan gets away to Pennsylvania anytime she can. Jason and Moyra set up home in Hoboken in a committed way. Andrea just invested in a place on the Lower East Side—she's an anomaly. Richard and Daniel made the move to the Slope . . . And so on. I won't bore you with the real estate issues of my friends. I'm looking for an answer to the question that everyone I know faces: why am I still here? I can live somewhere else much better for much cheaper. It seemed that New York was once hospitable to artists and the like. Now we know that's not the case. I stay around for my friends, because of the relationships I've formed—that's what most say.

Me: I'm going to stick around and watch it all rot. I want to be like Gibbon and document the decline. I want to be a poet of decay. But is New York dying, or is it me who's on his way out, harboring an evil wish to take it all with me? If I must end, must this end too? Given all the subjective concerns clouding my objectivity, listed haphazardly above, I can't know. It seems conceivable that a shift will occur. New York City cannot be the capital in the next century. Some say it will form somewhere on the Pacific rim—Tokyo, Hong Kong, Singapore. Others, presupposing the success of a unified European economy, have their money on Berlin. A few think that the center will remain in a United States that exists as part of an alliance with all the countries making up the Americas. The projections for Africa are not hopeful.

Too late for me. I won't be around to move to the next center. The content of my life is dissipation. I don't think the cracks in the viaducts are figments of my imagination. The roads are verifiably in disrepair. Still, people will continue to strive. More tall buildings will be built for conglomerates that go bankrupt. The kids will continue to invent scenes and the grown-ups will follow. The art world will move to Chelsea, then fracture and move again . . . Keep in mind that Manhattan is an island. It's an ideal, an aspiration, and like all absolute horizons it can never really exist. Not as a pure state of limitlessness.

I was born in the capital of the twentieth century. Rather, in Queens. Close enough to it to make the passage to the world's center safely. Compared to the journey my forebearers endured, it was easy. I am the last of my kin remaining in these parts. The rest have followed a southerly course continuing their Diaspora. I remain here, the last vestige of old world yearning. My grandfather hates Manhattan. For the last twenty-five years of his work life he labored in the basement of the Linden Clock Factory on Broadway and Twenty-Fifth. It's no wonder why he sought out the warmth of the sun in his retirement. For my grandfather, Manhattan was a job.

For me it was an exploration. My first excursion into the city was the yearly school trip for borough kids—a safari to the Museum of Natural History. Among the halls, the exhibits, the dioramas, the mammals of the sea provoked awe. I was eight when I first looked up in horror at the life-size whale suspended from the ceiling. It had a diminishing effect on me. I feared that it would fall. How can the roof suspend what takes an entire ocean to float? . . . What the whale was to Ahab, has been hinted; what, at times, he was to me, as yet remains unsaid . . . Am I Ishmael or Jonah? Do I hunt the whale, or has it swallowed me whole? Is the choice to remain in Manhattan a blind commitment to a quest borne on one of the many waves of immigration? Or, is it not a choice at all? Am I a captive of the beast?

Chapter 8
New York Was Yesterday

[A Conversation with Delmore Schwartz]

A twentieth-century Job, the writer Delmore Schwartz suffered the trials of both critical acclaim and crushing failure. Dead for over thirty years, Schwartz remains brilliant and manic depressive. I recently caught up with the man in a run-down Times Square hotel. A fresh shave and a clean but tattered suit weren't enough to cover the obviously depleted state of this literary genius. Pieces of toilet paper hung from his chin, secured by red blood stains. His teeth were yellowed and his finger tips were stained to match. He smelled. None of these things lessened the awe with which I approached the author of "In Dreams Begin Responsibilities." After we removed the sanitary wrapping off the hotel glasses, we sat down to chat over a few shots from the bottle of Johnnie Walker Red that the writer kept in the night table next to the bed for just such an occasion.

Delmore Schwartz: I was a good person but I expected too much from other people and then I turned mean.
Gregg Bordowitz: What did you want from others?
DS: Unconditional love. A child should receive that from his parents. If he doesn't when he's young, he'll yearn for it the rest of his life. When you're an adult it's too late. Everyone expects something from the ones they love. Adults must give love to get love . . . Listen young fella, I'm sure you didn't come here to talk like this. What do you want from me?
GB: Well, I'd like to talk about anything you want. I think you're a brilliant writer. *Pause. My compliment doesn't move him. Schwartz's eyes are glassy. He sips his drink slowly so as not to dribble.* Uh, I'm writing a column for an art journal about New York City, and I wanted to get your thoughts about the city.
DS: An art journal. What's your politics?

GB: Uh, well . . .
DS: My colleagues and I were struggling to keep our faith both in writing and in socialism. Both held out the potential for bettering the world. Maintaining faith in either enterprise was difficult at the time. Many of our ideals could not survive the revelations concerning Stalin. More than that. Much of modern literature wasn't concerned with preserving or recasting

great traditions. Me, I wanted to be the Jewish-American Shakespeare. I wrote a whole novel in verse. Have you read it?

GB: No, it's not in print so it's very difficult to find.

DS: Do you know where the library is? It's the big building with lions in front only a few blocks from here.

GB: I've read your stories and poems many times.

DS: Thanks . . . for nothing. What do you want, a medal? You think you can come here and what and what!? Why did you come here?

GB: I want to know if you think there's any hope for New York. Do you think it's still a town where a young guy can make his future?

DS: How the hell should I know? I've been dead longer than you've been living. Listen, boychik, it's sad that you came here. What do I have to offer you? Even when I was alive I didn't cope well. I went to the movies instead.

GB: Today, life is a very rough approximation of the movies.

DS: It's always been that way. What do you think? It was better when I was alive? No. It was the same. Isn't it the same now? I don't know. You tell me. You tell me. What's different? You're alive. You tell me.

GB: The Soviet Union doesn't exist anymore.

DS: This is news? The Soviet Union died during my lifetime. What else?

GB: Today, I can write a letter and send it, electronically, to almost anywhere in the world in a matter of seconds. The words never have to touch paper.

DS: What's it say?

GB: What?

DS: This letter? What's it say?

GB: I don't know, anything, I guess.

DS: Then it doesn't matter how fast it gets there. Look, I lived through the Depression and then a war and this is not to mention my personal problems. I'm the first generation of my people born here. I went to college. I became a very famous poet. And I died. I died here. Washed-up. Unknown. Not appreciated. So don't talk to me about a future. I didn't make my future in this city. I died in this city. I could have lived in Poughkeepsie for all it mattered. When I was young I had a future, but as I grew older my past continually ate my future. What do you do? Are you a writer?

GB: No, I'm a filmmaker.

DS: A filmmaker. Now that's an art form with a future. I love the movies.

GB: I'm losing interest in the movies. More movies are being made now than ever before. You can't imagine how many.

DS: It doesn't matter how many movies there are in the world. There is always room for one more good movie. Just worry about making a good movie. You want some advice? You must make a movie that faces up to the disappointments in your life. More than that, your movie must stand up to the false promises of the future without giving up hope.

GB: Hope?

DS: Yes, hope. Don't you know what hope is? It's a yearning to be free of the pain inflicted on us by our pasts. I thought you said you read my stories. If you become reconciled to your past, you give up on your future. This is a very complicated business. There's no way to become reconciled to the past without accepting the present. If you're living a miserable present, then accepting it will kill you. And you seem miserable.

GB: I do?

DS: Why else would you be inside drinking with a corpse on a nice day like this?

GB: The dead are better company than the living.

DS: We're not a threat. We're dead. We can't compete. You think if I was alive I'd be sitting around here moaning with you? No, I'd be writing or seeing a movie. Reading a paper. I can't do these things anymore because memory has fixed me in this hotel with the same damn bottle of scotch that never runs out. I can drink and drink, but I don't get drunk and I have to suffer whiners like you who beat a path to my door to worship at the altar of despair. You, pathological mourners who have made a cult out of melancholy.

GB: I'm melancholic? When's the last time you read your work? I've wept reading your stories.

DS: Sure. Sure. I was a mess, but I wrote funny pieces too. Have you read those?

GB: Those short things? Now you listen. Your funny pieces weren't so funny. Your humor usually revolved around the premise of defeat. Or, you thought it was amusing to reduce a concept like existentialism to the act of taking a bath. The laughter in these pieces was forced and the most evident characteristic of the writing was a strong sense of resignation and defeat.

DS: A critic? Tell me, Mr. Big Shot Filmmaker who doesn't write but has a column in a pisher ART journal. What have you accomplished?

GB: Nothing. I don't feel like I've accomplished anything.

DS: When I was twenty-four I owned the world. I was called the voice of my generation. I had chutzpah. Are you famous?

GB: No. I enjoy a small measure of provincial notoriety.

DS: Fame is a wonderful thing, but only an infinitesimal number of the planet's population will achieve true universal fame like . . . Marilyn Monroe. If this is true, why should American culture, a democratic culture, admire the few recognizably special among us? Almost everybody can be recognized by their nearest and dearest—in a crowd, in the morgue, or in a police line-up. Why strive for any more recognition than that? Everyone knows deep down that the best you can hope for is a decent photo on your driver's license.

GB: You had fame. You were known and well respected.

DS: That and a token got me on the subway. Fame ruined me.

Figure 8.2 Zoe Leonard, "Two Chairs." © Zoe Leonard, from an ongoing series begun in 1998.

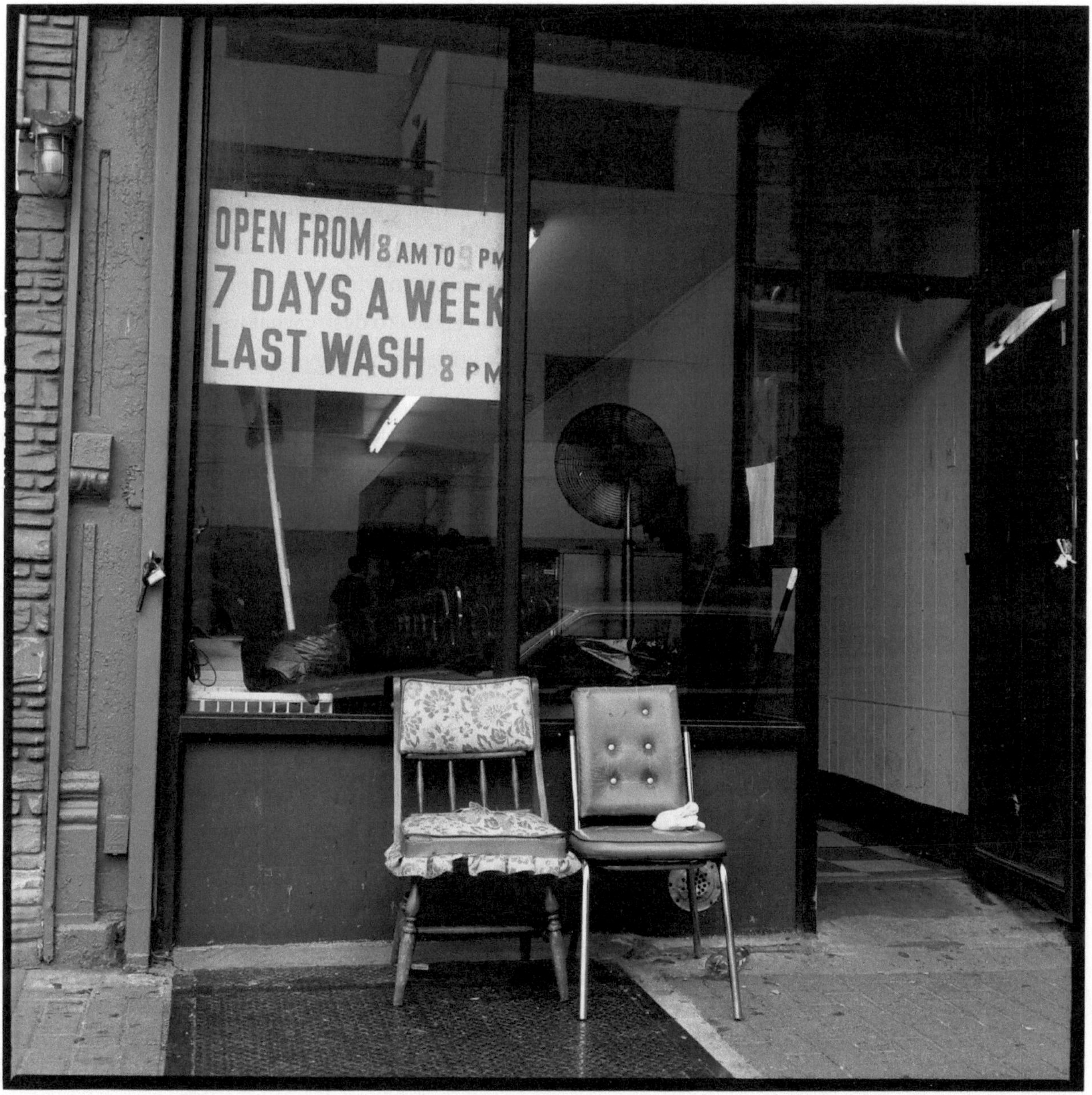
OPEN FROM 8 AM TO 9 PM
7 DAYS A WEEK
LAST WASH 8 PM

GB: It costs a dollar fifty now.

DS: What?

GB: The subway.

DS: That's a crime.

GB: You weren't ever a wealthy man.

DS: The best efforts of the twentieth century were devoted to equal distribution of wealth. But revolutionaries never understand the motivation behind greed. Fame and wealth are ideals to inspire us. Without such motivation where would we be? If we don't learn to desire what we can't have at the earliest possible age we won't budge from the cradle. Civilization could cease to exist because of crib death. We need the shiny creatures dangled just beyond our reach. Listen, most of us fail in our lifetime. We do not succeed according to the terms of success honored in our society. The question is: when so much of what so many of us achieve fails to hit the high mark intended, when all around us market and social forces demand compromise, why are failure and mediocrity despised?

GB: That's a joke right? You're kidding?

DS: You don't have my sense of humor. I'm completely serious and that's what's funny.

Chapter 8

New York Was Yesterday

[Renew Our Days]

I saw a documentary on television about the Yiddish language newspaper the *Forward.* An elderly man, a long-time editor of the paper, talked about a series of articles that appeared in the early part of the century, instructing newly arrived immigrants how to behave in the large crowds on New

York City streets. If you bump into someone on the street, say "Excuse me" and continue on. If someone steps on your toe at the market, don't make a fuss, it was probably an accident. Cover your mouth when you cough in public and so on. I don't know who these instructions were intended to benefit, but I assume they addressed immigrants from rural Eastern Europe and Russia, like some of my family.

In "On Some Motifs in Baudelaire" Walter Benjamin notes that "Fear, revulsion, and horror were the emotions which the big city crowd aroused in those who first observed it." Benjamin cites Edgar Allan Poe's short story "The Man of the Crowd." Poe observes, according to Benjamin, that the crowd "has something barbaric; discipline just barely manages to tame it." In the story, a man who is recuperating from a serious illness ventures out into the city after a long convalescence. He sits in a coffee-house staring out of the window, transfixed for hours by the endless stream of humanity.

> With my brow to the glass, I was thus occupied scrutinizing the mob, when suddenly there came into view a countenance (that of a decrepit old man, some sixty-five years of age)—a countenance which at once arrested and absorbed my whole attention, on account of the absolute idiosyncrasy of its expression.

Unable to let the old man out of sight, overcome by a desire "to know more of him," the protagonist grabs his coat and runs after the mysterious man, who leads him on a horrifying journey. The man of the crowd wanders aimlessly through the city streets. He doesn't care about the direction of his walking. He is lost to the city, a casualty of design. The movement of his gait is an oscillation independent of the body. The atmosphere swirls around his figure. Sounds and smells travel through the air fanned by his limbs. Wherever he finds himself, uptown or downtown, underground or above, he is always in motion. He can never arrive at a destination because his role as a pedestrian is a terminal condition.

Following the old man all night until the evening of the next day, the protagonist is finally exhausted by his doppelgänger's deviations—

> And, as shades of the second evening came on, I grew wearied unto death, and, stopping fully in front of the wanderer, gazed at him steadfastly in the face. He noticed me not, but resumed his solemn walk, while I, ceasing to follow, remained absorbed in contemplation. "This old man," I said at length, "is the type and the genius of deep crime."

Today, Poe's man of the crowd is embodied in the figure of a young muscular man on a Stairmaster. The urban rambler is driven into the new century on his chariot—the Stairmaster. It's the latest advance in treadmill technology. You've seen him staring blankly out of the large glass windows of a store-front gym, marching among the ranks of the physically fit, enveloped in the mood of his music entering his ears through the headphones of a Walkman strapped to his side. From his stationary position, ascending in place, he looks down on the passing crowds while excelling far above their pedestrian efforts. Nothing as aimless as a walk could possibly transport today's urban wanderer to where he aspires. He wants to advance, to climb high, to reach new levels. A line drawing of peaks and valleys charts his path forward on a monitor mounted to the frame of the marvelous contraption. His trajectory is not bound by any geographical limit. The trek is potentially infinite. The fitness machine can outlast any user. As one mortal drops another waits in line to take his place. An end is never reached.

In the future, the Stairmaster will be the preferred mode of travel. It will be a required appliance in every home. This prediction is based on the most current speculations about urban sprawl. Eventually, the city will spread out to cover the earth. The entire planet will become an urban entity. Travel will remain an essential concept, but the effort of travel will become unnecessary. The explanation for this is mathematical. Space is no longer measured in quantities of distance but in units of time. Rate of speed bears only a symbolic relation to miles, much as money now only vaguely refers to the gold standard. Think about frequent flier miles. Distance has become a unit of measure to be sold and traded like quantities of dollars to be credited—or debited—from our money card accounts. The value of these units will decrease when the travel industry is no longer a going concern. When the world is one city, every place will look the same as everywhere else. The desire to go anywhere will no longer excite even the most melancholy soul. (Travel was once considered *the* cure for melancholia.) What will people do with their time once space is no longer part of the equation? Zeno's paradox will become the governing law of physics on Earth: Motion is impossible. If space is infinitely divisible, any finite distance must, allegedly, consist in an infinite number of points; and as everybody knows, it is impossible to reach the end of an infinite series of operations in a finite time. For example, say that you're running to catch a bus. Before you reach the bus, you must reach the halfway point between you and the bus. Before you reach that, you must reach the halfway point to it. I never take the bus.

I ride the subway. A glimmer of light illuminates the track moments before the subway appears. When it comes, it's a miracle. I may be running late for an appointment but when I step into the subway car I am always not-yet-late. The train relinquishes me of all responsibility. How can I get there any faster?

Some commuters sleep through the tunnels, gathering strength for the efforts that await their arrival. Others read books studying for the tests that lie ahead. Many read newspapers. Ernst Bloch wrote that the value of today's newspaper is greatly exaggerated and the value of yesterday's news is underestimated. He thought that a liberating piece of news was likely to come from an old paper. Years ago, I rode the subway with my grandfather from Manhattan back to Queens. He was returning home after a long day's work. I asked him why he read the *Daily News* and not the *New York Times.* I said that the *Times* gives much more information than the *News.* His reply: "I don't need to know that much."

My grandfather's parents fled the pogroms to settle in Jewish slums. He inherited their disappointment and paranoia. I did not. Growing up in Queens during the seventies I enjoyed a model experience of multiculturalism. I knew I was a Jew. Others viewed me as Jewish and I viewed others variously as Irish, Puerto Rican, black, Italian, and Korean—all groups well represented in my neighborhood. Each group had its own seemingly indissoluble identity, yet we coexisted. We all understood ourselves to be different from each other and at the same time we had an understanding of ourselves as a neighborhood. We coped with our diversity. There were tensions between groups but it was possible to have close relationships across ethnic boundaries. Class played an important role, because we were all from working families facing the same material conditions. We all shared lower middle class aspirations.

We climbed. We scaled for a better purchase. I clambered alongside my fellow grade school graduates from P.S. 186. Rather than accept what I felt to be my sentence—manual labor at minimum wage—I succeeded on to the page. Writing is climbing for some. Each word you see before you is a step in a direction away from an undesirable conclusion. Each step feels like progress upward, but writing is an inevitable descent. So is reading.

Every word leads to the bottom of the page. This text is an exercise contraption. It's an exhausting simulation of forward movement.

In drawing a line of distinction between a people and a mob, we shall find that a people aroused to action are a mob, and that a mob trying to think, subside into a people. —Edgar Allan Poe, "The Southern Messenger," June 1849[1]

In eighteenth-century England the unregulated cost of foodstuffs often resulted in spontaneous actions by the mob. E. P. Thompson documented how the English working class developed out of this history of rebellions: "Food riots were sometimes uproarious, like the 'Great Cheese Riot' at Nottingham's Goose Fair in 1764, when whole cheeses were rolled down the streets."[2]

The AIDS Coalition to Unleash Power used to stage rebellions over the high cost of drugs. The first was on Wall Street in March of '87. Later in the movement, concerns about drug costs gave rise to the demand that People with AIDS control the entire drug research agenda. The lasting contribution of the AIDS activist movement is the principle that people with a disease should be directly involved in making decisions that affect care and treatment. Into the history of what new class will this contribution be recorded? Or, is it part of the history of a class politics in decline?

1. Edgar Allen Poe, *The Book of Poe,* ed. Addison Hibbard (Garden City, New York: Doubleday, Doran, 1929), p. 154.
2. E. P. Thompson, *The Making of the English Working Class* (New York: Vintage Books, 1963), p. 64.

Often I recognize the familiar faces of dead friends among the crowd. Enormous numbers of people can't fill the void of a significant loss. The isolation one feels among the crowd is not the same as the solitary enterprise of the treadmill. Walking forward through the city one is forced to face the other. I am unknown to you as you are unknown to me. What makes us strangers to each other makes us recognizable to ourselves. The simple physical law that no two bodies can occupy the same space at the same time translates into an ethical principle—each has the same value as the other.

[A Solemn Assembly]

Daniel was over for the supper the other night and the table conversation occasioned the opportunity for him to sing his old school song for us, with lyrics by William Blake:

Bring me my bow of burning gold
Bring me my arrows of desire
Bring me my spear; O clouds unfold!
Bring me my Chariot of Fire.
I will not cease from mental fight
Nor shall my sword sleep in my hand
Till we have built Jerusalem . . .

I asked him if his school was Zionist. He laughed. "No," he corrected, "Jerusalem as an ideal."

Jerusalem—the city at the center of the four points of the compass, the navel of the world. Yes, an ideal. Jerusalem has always represented the ideal of an international city and now that the time for nations is over, at the end of the twentieth century, this ideal is necessary. Jerusalem could be a city which belonged to no nation, truly a city of the world. Of course, the reality is sobering: so many have laid claim to Jerusalem that it continues to be one of the most contested sites in the world. Jerusalem should become a multinational municipality. What governing body could administer the daily business of such a place? I am not a politician, but an idealist. The possibility of a self-governed, polyglot, multiracial, multiethnic, nondenominational, secular cosmopolis is my idea of heaven on earth.

At supper, Daniel and I discussed Middle East politics until our attention was taken by Jesus across the table, who loudly introduced a topic into discussion: the end of the rent control rebellion. We were all saddened by the failure of the rebellion. The remains of the barricades had been cleared away by sanitation workers. The city, in its drive to put down all resistance, paid overtime for the extra manpower to clean up the mess. Jesus has a new term—*Parisization*—to describe the government's efforts to remove all poverty from the island of Manhattan itself and relegate the working populations to the outer boroughs, where they can easily travel to the city's center to man the shops, drive the taxis, and clean the homes.

Jesus held the table's attention with a sneer across his face, "No one poor lives in Paris proper. When I visit major European cities I always stay in a suburb because the people I visit are of roughly the same economic standing, within their respective economies, as I am. Artists, intellectuals, bohemians, live near—but not in—the city. New York will be the same. Manhattan will eventually be an island for the rich. Bad news for the young artists who continue to arrive daily. It is no longer possible to live poor and make art in New York City. One might as well wear a beret, move to Paris, and paint Cubist canvases. The idea of New York as a vital artistic laboratory is as moribund, as historical, as Paris, capital of the nineteenth century." We all laughed bitterly.

At first the rebellion didn't seem possible. Who could have imagined? The "man-on-the-street" interviews presented on the local news seemed to confirm—enforce—the opinion that rent control was an archaic system that unfairly benefited the few. They contended that the system prevented the equitable formulation of prices for rentals, co-ops, and condos.

Jesus, a master logician, Socratically teased the dinner party: "Let us suppose that (a) rent control is an archaic system that unfairly benefits only a small group of people, not all of whom are poor or in need of assistance. Yes, let's assume that, too. If (a) is true then (b) a universal application of rent control throughout New York City would fairly ensure that everyone had decent housing. Thus (c) rent control isn't the problem. Rather, the housing market is unfairly structured. It was the owners of real estate who first advanced the assertion that rent control is unfair."

We all nodded in agreement with Jesus' flawless reasoning. The core constituencies of the rebellion had been the elderly, the infirm, and the poor. Even the house-bound were wheeled out, after years of confinement, by family, friends, and live-in nurses to participate in the actions. The Upper West Side was closed off to all traffic. The rent control activists erected barricades of garbage, old furniture, and cars. They held strong for no less than three days. The biggest surprise was that their downfall was not at the hands of truncheon-wielding cops or burly sanitation workers. Armies of two-income couples in their thirties, mostly heterosexual, but with a noticeable contingent of lesbian and gay parents, organized into columns using baby carriages as battering rams and broke the barricades in an afternoon. The landlords held up the rear of the reactionary forces shouting promises of paint jobs and new appliances to inspire the mob. The forces for rent control could not withstand the assault from waves of well-dressed parents wearing the regulation office casual wear equipped with the latest in athletic foot gear.

Appalled at the spectacle of the citizenry at war with itself over real estate, the State Senate is entertaining legislation that will phase out rent control slowly, so that those who can remember that the State once assumed a role in providing affordable housing to the poor will no longer be alive to remind the next generation that housing is a right. New York will be a great place to raise kids, an environment devoid of the shabbily dressed, the ill-smelling, the foul-mouthed, the elderly, the sick, the queer, the fun, the fearless, the inspired, the creative. A New York without New Yorkers—an ideal of a sort. All of us at the supper felt gloomy about the prospects of the future. We sensed that something was coming to an end.

Daniel reintroduced the subject of Jerusalem to the table: "The Israeli government is building houses, claiming land, creating facts in territories owned by the wind, the rocks, in the name of a corrupt sectarian ideal." No one had anything to offer in response. Returning to the issue of rent control, I wondered aloud if we could not give a name to the sectarian forces inflicting violence in the rent control struggles? Peter smartly offered that class warfare was once the term used to describe such confrontations. Just then Judas choked on some matzoh and Jesus had to pound on his back with his fist. Judas drew in air sharply as the color returned to his face. We all laughed nervously and Miriam asked who among us would like some decaf.

The wine had dulled our senses, the coherence of our arguments declined as our voices rose. The table's discussion degenerated into babel, many small arguments competing. The mood for group discussion was finally lost after dessert when each one of us muttered the benedictions to ourselves. I closed my eyes mumbling nonsense, appearing to pray, waiting for someone else to finish first, and so ended the supper.

Our ties to beings and things are so fragile they often break without us noticing.

A breath, a glance, a sign, and sometimes just confiding a shadow: such is, roughly, the original nature of our ties.

If our ties are eternal, it is because they are divine.

You try to be free through writing. How wrong. Every word unveils another tie. —Reb Leca in Edmond Jabès, The Book of Questions[1]

Chapter 8

New York Was Yesterday

Dear Reader,

I have a confession to make. I've lied. Oh, I've lied more than once within these pages but the margins can only contain one admission for the moment. A journal can't sustain the many rents full disclosure would abuse

1. Edmond Jabès, *The Book of Questions,* trans. Rosemarie Waldrop (Middletown: Wesleyan University Press, 1976), p. 37.

upon its spine. And I will not reduce to pulp the body upon which my life feeds. The book is the only horizon I have left to follow.

In spite of my promise—to myself with you as my witness (you can't escape blame, for I don't exist without you; isn't this an act of collusion?)—to remain in New York as a chronicler of its passing, I have abjured my morbid responsibilities and staked a claim in another once-great American city.

You keep your New York joys
I'm going to Illinois, just as fast as I can

Count Basie wrote the score, and we have but to listen.

Good-bye, farewell, I'm a see you later
Going to Chicago, sorry but I can't take you

In the tune, New York breaks the heart and Chicago is the line of retreat. New York's a cruel lover. It's true. New York doesn't care whether you live or die, whether you stay or leave, even if you pull down six figures, drive an off-road, and enjoy eating business-class cuisine in cavernous cafeterias of dubious design.

You can't really leave. New York is everywhere and nowadays anywhere can be New York. America is a parking-lot-drive-in-Hollywood-Hard-Rock-Cafe with high priced-soilent green food ground from the bones of old starlets. And so too Chicago is a corruption of our dreams. It all comes down to Queens. I never left. Standing now on the corner of Augusta and Western looking over the roofs of two- and three-story houses, one can see the John Hancock Center, "one of three giants that dominate the late-twentieth-century Chicago skyline" (according to the American

Institute of Architects Guide). The skyline is a competition among boasting first-person pronouns that dominate a landscape of surrounding conjunctions. I will now inhabit the flatlands of endless deferral. The dream deferred *is* the dream and the dream's realization is a poor copy of the borough's designs. Here the whole city is one sprawling borough. I embrace the borough, lost to the sprawl, my forty days and forty nights, a wandering. Here urban mystery is found haunting abandoned industrial spaces. (No more empty space in New York, every inch is instrumentalized toward the dead ends of capital.) "Chicago Is Dying" (too) screamed a poster wheat-pasted under the El at Damen and Milwaukee, protesting the gentrification that will surely swallow this metropolis, albeit at a slower pace. New York cooks faster because Manhattan's flame burns incandescent. That's central heating. Here, the heat's more elusive. The city's been burned down before.

Nelson Algren is my spiritual sponsor in "The City on the Make"—

> Yet if you've tried New York for size and put in a stint in Paris, lived long enough in New Orleans to get the feel of the docks and belonged to old Marseilles awhile, if the streets of Naples have warmed you and those of London have chilled you, if you've seen the terrible green-grey African light moving low over the Sahara or even passed hurriedly through Cincinnati—then Chicago is your boy at last and you can say it and make it stick.[2]

Shy-town is funky. The buildings on my block are not of uniform design. Each is a slightly different variant of a model long lost to memory, if an original ever existed. My new address is on Iowa Street. Every time I

2. Nelson Algren, *City on the Make* (Chicago: University of Chicago Press, 1987), p. 42.

find my way home I arrive somewhere else. Unmoored, unmasked, unmanned, going horizontal and sprawling, I'm a threat to the landscape, like Cézanne who thought each part was as important as any other. The surface is sheer and perilous. I'll tumble off the table, yet.

When you see me passin', hang your head and cry.

Enough with the melancholic contrivances and the boohoohoo over yesterday. The great American city is as unattainable as the great American novel. The figure of the city itself is about as archival as a trade paperback whose spine is meant to be broken by mass transit consumption. So enough with the absent father and the castrating mother. So what? Enough with the tribal warfare and blood grudges of the Holy Land. Enough wailing. Enough diaspora. We're lost whether we move or stay. Lost is our condition.

Hurry, hurry down sunshine and see what tomorrow brings
Well the sun went down and tomorrow brought us rain.

Having unpacked my library, I have rediscovered books that I had forgotten or never bothered to read. Among them John Cage's writings. One fine example of his mesostic form is "25 Mesostics Re and Not Re Mark Tobey" in which he used the name of his friend, the painter Mark Tobey, as the basis for the poem's stanzas.[3] For example, the poem begins:

3. John Cage, "25 Mesostics Re and Not Re Mark Tobey." *Postmodern American Poetry: A Norton Anthology,* ed. Paul Hoover (New York and London: W. W. Norton, 1994), 18–21.

it was i**M**possible
to do **A**nything
the doo**R**
was loc**K**ed

Another stanza that I like:

you can find ou**T**
what kind **O**f art is up to the minute
By visiting
th**E** head office
of a successful advertising compan**Y**

Inspired by Cage's wordplay, his methods using chance operations and his commitment against expressivity, I decided to rethink the "Basic Concepts" as they are listed in the table of contents in Raymond Williams's *Marxism and Literature* (Oxford Univ. Press, 1977).

Clearly
yo**U**
Laugh
Too
rel**U**ctantly
Revolutionary
Enthusiasts

Life
b**A**lances
upo**N**

uG**G**ly

bea**U**ty

And

Glorious

Evil

too **L**ate

for h**I**story

our cen**T**ury

is **E**mptied

of **R**esources

All our

Texts

red**U**ced

to **R**ags

and cind**E**rs

l**I**es

not free**D**om

p**E**rpetrated by us

up**O**n us

with zea**L** we

deny f**O**rm

and despite our **G**ood intentions

we **Y**ield to an impoverishing content

Chicago is my retreat. Here among my books and compact discs, I hide from the winter's cold convictions. Rereading a book is like visiting an old friend whose life has continued along its own trajectory. Ideas do not age so much as they mature. There are many more nuances than I could see in my ignorant self-absorbed youth. I spend my days in the Midwest pondering what Gertrude Stein meant when she said that "A sentence is not emotional a paragraph is." I listen to Lambert, Hendricks and Ross, Sonny Stitt and Brother Jack McDuff, Morton Feldman, the Kronos Quartet, Sonic Youth and STEREOLAB. Plus, I'm learning how to cook. Cooking is poetry pursued by other means. As you can see I've been cooking a lot with the old recipes to serve new dishes. The following was written using the basic recipe for borscht from *The Joy of Cooking*, substituting each ingredient with a word taken at random from the dictionary. I accepted every choice chance made.

Peel and chop until very fine:
    1/2 cup fun
    1 cup illogicality
    2 cups curtain
Barely cover these ingredients with boiling water.
Simmer gently, covered for about 20 minutes. Add and simmer for 15 minutes more:
    1 tablespoon ideal
    2 cups stolidity or other state of affairs
    1 cup very finely shredded secret
    1 tablespoon umbra
Place in bowls. Add to each serving:
    1 tablespoon of cultured deoxyribonucleic acid
mixed with:
    Grated soliloquy
    correct seasoning
and serve hot or cold with:
    nought

Figure 8.3 Zoe Leonard, "TV Repair Shop." © Zoe Leonard, from an ongoing series begun in 1998.

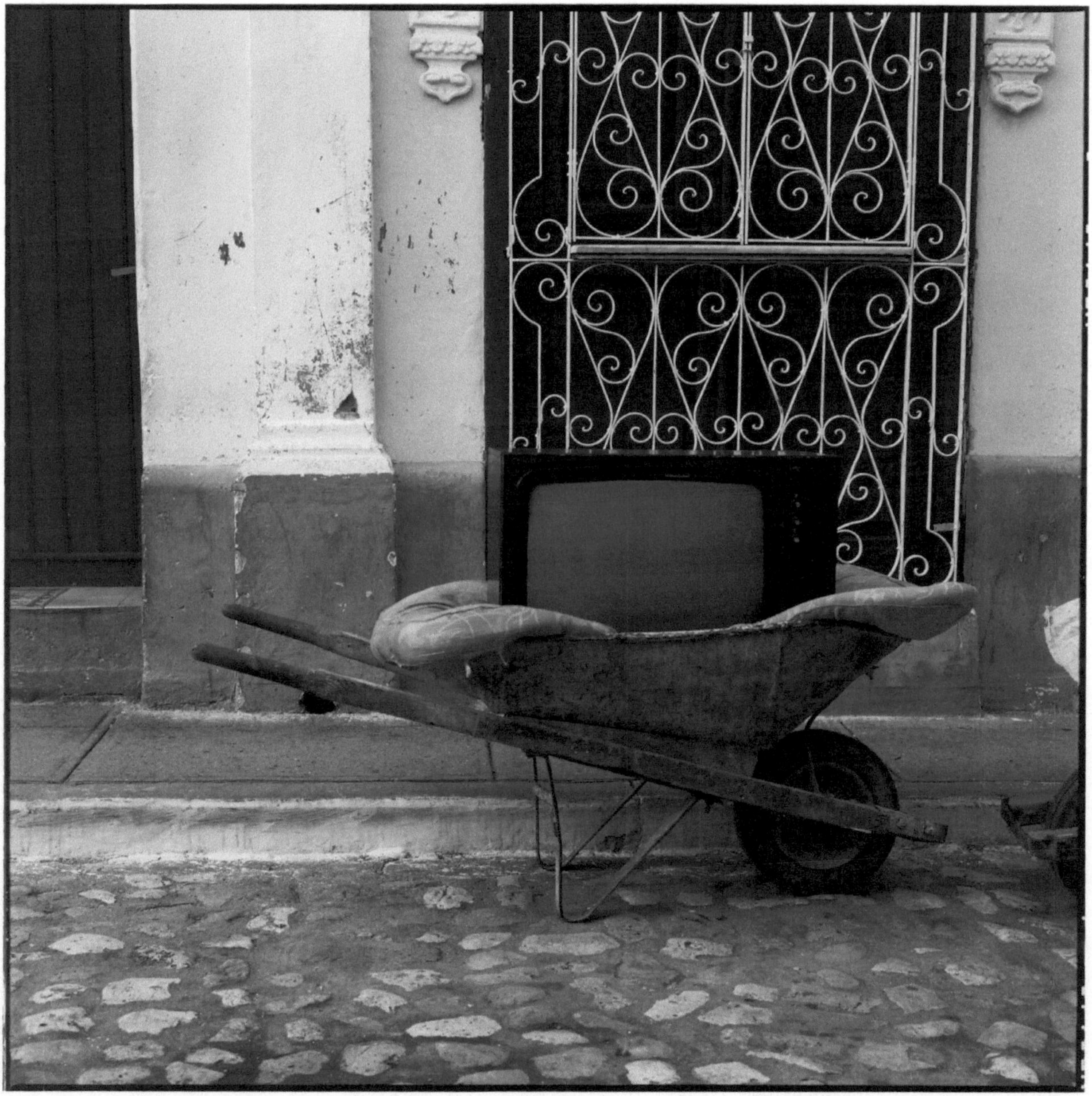

Figure 8.4 Zoe Leonard, "Pharmacy." © Zoe Leonard, from an ongoing series begun in 1998.

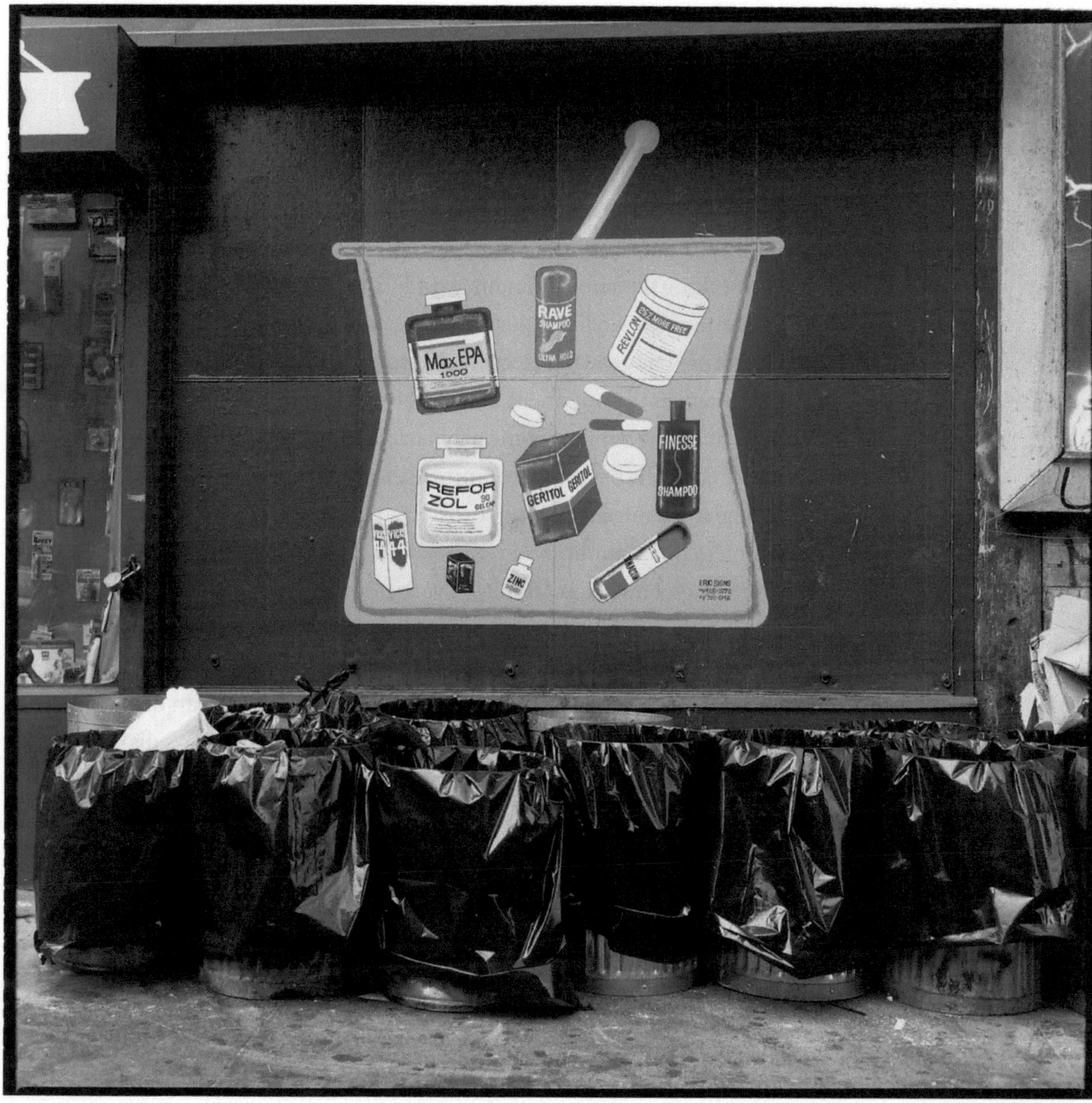
Max EPA
1000
RAVE
SHAMPOO
ULTRA HOLD
REVLON
25% MORE FREE
FINESSE
SHAMPOO
REFOR
ZOL
90
GEL CAP
GERITOL
GERITOL
VICKS
44
ZINC

A filling diet. That's why I walk around the neighborhood from Ukrainian Village to Wicker Park and back. The day is cloudless. The sky is a cantilever projecting far beyond the supporting wall of the city's skyline. In the summer, the heat rises from the prairies. Once the temperature hit over 107 degrees. I'm going swimming. Lake Michigan might as well be an ocean, you can't see the other side. Isn't the illusion of infinity the same thing as infinity? I may live until I'm forty and I don't want to stay in the same place, thinking the same thoughts, wondering the same things about a life that I presumed over, like a talentless sports team forced to play out the time. The score has grown obscenely disproportionate to the measure of creativity. It favors the opponent of Eros. Loss is assured. Regardless, I don't want to sit on the bench. Let me play, coach. How much damage can I do? Sports, specifically basketball, dominate the nightly news in Chicago, like the way the stock market controls broadcasts in New York. Every town has something to boast about.

Oh, New York. I miss you. In spite of your boorish arrogance. You are the alpha and omega of the urban religion. When will your power over me diminish? Even at your most vulgar you retain your balance. You know how to hold your liquor, New York. And I, a hopeless romantic, can only break free by denigrating you the way I demonize an old lover who's disappointed and forgotten me like yesterday's news.

Dear reader, I may have left New York, but I have not abandoned you. Though I have moved base camp to the foot of a new Olympus, I do not honor its gods. I remain a chronicler of waning ideals. The sun may set later in central time, but its flame extinguishes no less colorfully. With that in mind, let us not ignore the new surroundings. I am not devoting myself to the exhaustion of a theme simply to gratify my death drive. I'm searching for the new. For an alternative. And I will find it.

Faithfully yours,

9

Which Is More Powerful: The Word or the Idea?

Originally published as "Which Is More Powerful: The Word or the Idea?" in *Bodies of Resistance*, eds. Julia Bryan-Wilson and Barbara Hunt (New York: Visual AIDS and Real Artways, 2000), pp. 65–69. Minor revisions have been made for consistency.

Chapter 9
The Word or the Idea?

There is much to say and there is the feeling that the words do not yet exist to say what needs to be said.[1] That's the problem. Perhaps, it's not the words themselves but their correct combinations that will unlock the answers. "What's the question?" Gertrude Stein asked Alice B. Toklas on her deathbed. A question about a question is the closest thing to an answer our language has yet produced.

1. When Ray was in the hospital, his lover Tony occupied a bed down the hall. Both were terribly ill. The staff at the St. Vincent's AIDS ward were sensitive to the needs of

Alexander Pittleman is the name of this story's protagonist. He is a writer and he is afflicted with a disease that has no cure. There is no better hero of a story than the writer himself and there's no better authority on a disease than the diseased.

It is not yet light out. It is cold. Alexander is barely awake yet the first sentence of the day has already formed in his head. That's what woke him up:

Morning is liquid suspension.

He's standing in the kitchen. Waiting. Four quarter-size tablets of medicine slowly dissolve in a clear octagonal tumbler of water. Impatient to get to work, he can't wait any longer. He picks up a fork to stir the chalky solution; grinds the remaining solid matter against the side of the glass with the fork's tines; drinks it all down in one draught. It tastes like it tastes. He's used to it. That's all for now. It's forty-five minutes before he can take the remaining morning pills and eat breakfast. This is his morning, every day.

Mourning is a ritual, he thinks, muffling a laugh so as not to wake up the sleeper in the bedroom. She is sick. It's infuriating. It's not fair. Her illness upsets the order of the household; he is the sick one and she is the caretaker. That's childish. There it is. That's what it is. He knows it.

The most difficult thing in the world for him is responsibility for another's suffering. If he can't do anything to ease the other's suffering, he feels responsible for the suffering. A presumption of guilt precedes all of his thinking.

The next forty-five minutes will lapse slowly unless he does something to fill it with a content other than queasy hunger. He enters his office,

gay couples and offered to put them in the same room. Neither Ray nor Tony wanted this. Each couldn't bear to watch the other slowly die. During the period when they were hospitalized, I observed both weigh what they could give to each other against what each needed to do for himself. It was one of the most painful things I've ever had to witness. This fiction draws on that experience.

boots up the computer, clicks on the Word icon, types his first sentence onto the screen and stops. The next line refuses to come to mind. It's amazing how fast the well runs dry. He knows that it is best not to wait too long for the next line. He must turn his attention to something else.

The tarot deck is always within reach. Alexander shuffles the cards thoroughly. A quick read requires five cards. The first card drawn represents the situation of the reader. The Seven of Wands: a young man on a rocky hill grasps a flowering staff. Six other staves rise up against him. Here is a man holding his own against adversity with success and courage. But, the card is reversed; it is upside down, signifying perplexity, embarrassments, and anxiety. This is a warning against indecision.

Next: the Ace of Pentacles. A hand issuing forth from a cloud holds a pentacle, a disc with a five-pointed star on its center. Lilies grow in a garden below. The second card represents the situation or problem that the reader faces. Pentacles signify material concerns: money and fortune. The card is not reversed; the advantages of the card favor the reader.

The third card drawn represents the problems or difficulties the reader has facing his situation. The Eight of Cups, reversed. Eight golden goblets stacked neatly in the foreground. In the background, a man of dejected affect has turned his back on the cups; he is walking away. Streams, mountains and rocks lie before him. On the face of it, the meaning of the card is obvious: you have turned your back on material success for something higher. Reversed, this card could mean just the opposite: you've abandoned the spiritual for the material. This could portend great joy, partying and happiness. In this reading, with the Eight of Cups following the Ace of Pentacles (fending off adversity), the cards are saying that you are preoccupied with your material well-being. You are preoccupied to the extent that all of your energy is focused on your work. The work you're doing isn't what you want to be doing with your time.

Strengths or dominant aspects are the concerns of the fourth card drawn: the Page of Wands, reversed. The Page represents the eternal messenger. He stands tall. He's making a proclamation. In the background mounds in the shape of pyramids sit on the horizon. Are these mounds in the background burial mounds? Reversed, this card can mean bad news. Does the Page in this instance bring news of death? If so, is it the death of the reader (author), or someone else? Could this be a wake-up call? In this position of the reading the card and the news it delivers are strong factors in the final outcome.

The last card in this lay reveals the outcome: the card for Strength. It signifies fortitude, but it's reversed. (The number of reversed cards in this reading is significant: you're working through a lot of negativity here.) A woman is shown confidently closing a lion's mouth. The lion is subdued. Wild forces are tamed before this woman. The symbol of infinity floats above her head. For a consciousness that is aware of eternity, there are no obstacles, no resistances. Around her waist she wears a chain of flowers; nature is a light burden upon her figure, an adornment. The divinatory meaning of the card is apparent: spiritual power overcoming material power; or higher nature over carnal power (the lion is an aspect of passion). Reversed, the card suggests the domination of the material. It also suggests discord.

Facing adversity in the material world, the reader seeks comfort from bad news and indecision by turning his attention to material comforts. This direction is not entirely bad. It seems for the moment that the reader has control of the material conditions in his life. However, he must be aware that by favoring material comfort and security he's denying his passions. The reading warns of ill fortune to come if awareness of the eternal principle remains submerged. Unconscious.

This rings bells for Alex. He returns the five cards to the deck, shuffles it, and draws one more card. This card determines his course of action. He picks The World reversed. The World is the highest card in the deck; it holds the promise of nothing less than cosmic perfection (if one draws it right side up). In its reversed form The World warns against fear of change. It means that the earthbound spirit is attached to one place or profession and that's not good. Alex's spirit is slothful and stubborn. Nothing will change until he learns the lessons of past experiences.

It is difficult to perform a tarot reading for oneself. Not recommended.

An hour and a half has passed. Seven more pills to swallow and it's time for nourishing food substances: cereal in milk, toast, coffee and juice. A hacking cough knocks gently at the other side of the closed door of the bedroom. He stops eating. Should he check on her? Silence. He listens. Silence. Back to his cereal. The crunching sound inside his own skull plugs his ears. He can't hear her and he can't hear himself think. What's the next line to write? He's up two hours and it's taken him this long to dispense with medicines and breakfast. Now he can get down to some serious work. Alex returns to the desk.

It's quiet in the house. There's not a sound coming from the adjacent bedroom. His office, the kitchen and the bedroom are architecturally triangulated within the layout of the small house. This design suits him. Eat, sleep and work. That is the shape of his existence. Closing his eyes, he plots a point in the center of each of the three rooms. Eyes still closed he connects the dots to form a perfect equilateral triangle. His mind is wandering further and further away from the task at hand.

Morning is a liquid suspension.

The theme concerns dissolution. Dispersion. He is disappearing, sublating into the atmosphere. The weight-loss is noticeable. The mirror returns a cadaverous self-image. He's never been this thin. The doctor cannot tell him if the disease causes the wasting, or if it's a side effect of the drugs that are prolonging his life. Alex doesn't think the cause matters. He can see the veins in his arms and thighs. His belly button protrudes. His cheeks are sunken hollows. He is more afraid of appearing ill than feeling ill. His worst fear is realized: he is visibly, apparently ill. And he is ashamed of his narcissism. A problem of privilege. He remains relatively healthy. The monthly blood tests show no measurable trace of the killer virus. Yet, he is diabetic (probably another side effect of the drugs). His cholesterol is high. Death will come from one thing or another.

Morning and mourning are homonyms, calling to mind the beginning and the end. Alex likes that. The sound of retching from the room on the other side of the wall disturbs his concentration. He listens. Silence. What can he do? He feels powerless. Are words enough to save us? This thought occurs when the question of faith is posed. He only has faith in words. My illness. Her illness. The world is sick. Words can tell the truth as much as they can lie. So, why place one's faith in words? It is precisely because words can either be true or false that they deserve devotion. Meaning is not contingent on truth.

That's why he consults the tarot. He doesn't believe in a cosmic force that guides the hand. Alexander Pittleman is an atheist more often than he is not. Well-constructed rhetorical systems are fascinating: the tarot and the I Ching; astrology, numerology, psychoanalysis and modern scientific method (not so modern anymore). Medical science has prolonged his life, but no longer than the fragile ecology of a meaningful existence which prevents him daily from stepping in front of a subway train at rush hour.

He'll never do that. He never leaves the house anymore. There are ways to kill oneself in the house: household ways. He won't. He can't. He doesn't want to.

Perhaps he could kill her. Smother her incessant cough with a pillow. Alex shudders at the thought. God forgive me, he thinks. Since they both fell ill, a war over attention has divided the house. A distance as wide as the house separates them.

Does it matter who gave it to whom? He has the advantage. He has more resources. He has responded better to the drugs than she has. Her virus is multidrug-resistant.

Alexander pounds his palm against his head, gets up from the desk, circles the room, leaves the office, enters the kitchen. He opens the refrigerator and takes out a can of liquid nutritional supplement. Chocolate. The label instructs him to shake well. He pops the top and drinks the whole can. It's like motor oil: so thick. Immediately, he feels the stirs in his bowels. Alex runs to the toilet and manages to pull down his pajama pants just in time to release the explosion of gas and liquid that splatters the bowl, the seat, and the wall.

The bathroom is just off the kitchen. As he sits waiting for the episode to pass, Alex tries to imagine if and how the bathroom is part of the geometry of his mind's architectural design. Is the bathroom a necessary part of the daily machine, or is it an entirely independent structure? Obviously, it is connected to the daily enterprise in some primary way. It is fundamental. Alex redraws the floor plans of the house in his head. The shape of his existence is trapezoidal. This is not an elegant solution.

Seems like he's going to be on the toilet a while, so Alexander Pittleman reaches for a magazine. Leafing through the pages, he passes over images of cars and watches and shoes; a beautiful woman, a beautiful man, a bottle of liquor. All of these things elude his ownership and he will never possess them. He has copies of these things, but his things will always remain impoverished versions of the glossy ideals. One advertisement catches his attention. It advertises something that he must have. He cannot live without it. It's an ad for all the drugs he is currently taking. The five pharmaceutical companies that make the treatments for his disease have cooperated together on a ten-page supplement to extol the virtues of their products and to educate consumers about their treatment options.

On the cover of the advertising supplement there's a racing car speeding around a track coming toward the viewer. If one looks closely, one can see that the car is covered in decals. Each of the decals spells the name of one of the many drugs that comprise a full treatment regimen for people with Alex's disease. In the picture, crowds cheer the car from the bleachers surrounding the track. It's a sunny day. There are no other cars in sight. The pharmaceutical car is winning the race with a tremendous lead. In the foreground of the ad, there's a man standing, holding a checkered flag high above his head. The race is not yet over but the victory of corporate-fueled modern medicine seems assured.

This advertisement is too remarkable to be true. Alexander shakes his head with incredulity. Is it possible that I could be a winner? His hopes rise. Light-headed and feeling emptied of everything he's ingested today, Alex wipes himself clean.

The science of signs is perhaps one of the oldest. Interpreting the symbols in an allegory is perhaps the most difficult and enduring practice of the artist. If not the artist, then who? Who else can give meaning to these dark times? Alex is feeling grand. He understands the present. It's sad. These feelings are as fleeting as they are illusory, but they give him courage. The sense of comprehension is only a feeling, a sensation like a sugar rush. This assertion is easy to prove. It doesn't require biology. If you asked Alex to explain right now, this moment, what he thinks he understands, his high spirits would desert him. Let's not do that. Now that his courage is up, so too is his compassion.

Alex opens the door to the bedroom. He sticks his head in and softly whispers, "Hey, how are you feeling?" The room is hot. It smells of vomit. Alex remains on the threshold, his body half in and half out. No response. Alex inquires again in a loud stage whisper, "How are you feeling?"

"How do you think I'm feeling?" is the report from the darkness.

Alexander is confounded by that question. He knows the answer and he doesn't want to know it. Rather than face what he knows, he follows a seemingly unrelated line of thought. He closes the door, turns away and thinks to himself: the bedroom is a very strange place. It's where the day starts and where it concludes. It's where we retreat when we're ill. It's where we fuck and where we dream. Where whole novels are written and children are conceived. It's the locus of all we strive to avoid and everything we can't avoid. It's a void. And in this way, allowing the mind to wander, what seems at first to provoke a tangential escape route becomes a curved line that leads Alex back to what he struggles violently against.

There is no resolution to this story. The next line remains to be written. The author is not yet dead. Let's hope that with words we can conquer what for the time being we cannot cure; and that the meanings we make in our art do not dissipate our will to act. There are heights out of the reach of words, but no level reachable without them.

10

What the World Needs Now

South African HIVers Counter Doomsday Images with Profiles in Radical Courage

Originally published as "What the World Needs Now," *POZ* (May 2001): 40–42. Minor revisions have been made for consistency.

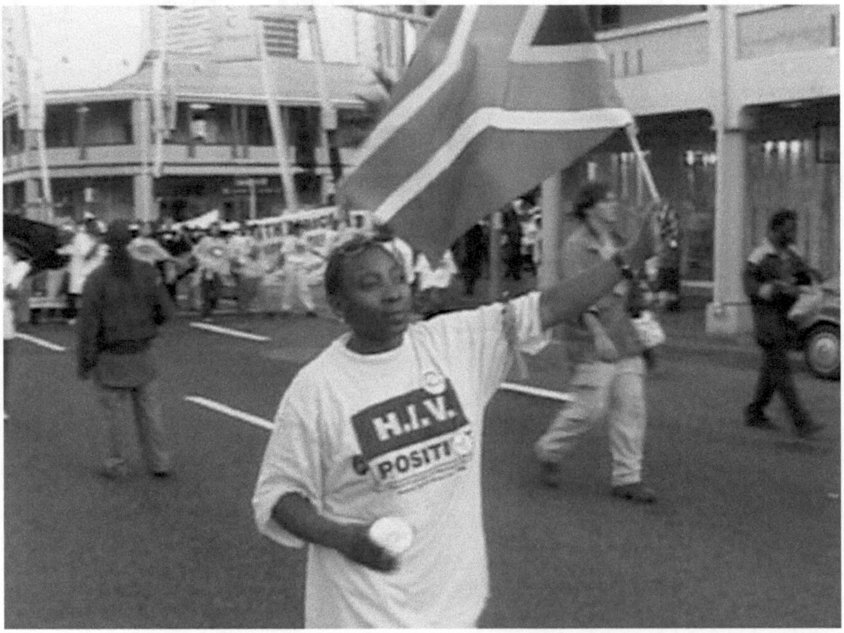

Figure 10.1 Protester in Durban, South Africa, 2000. From Gregg Bordowitz, *Habit*, 2001.

Chapter 10

What the World Needs Now

After the International AIDS Conference in Durban last July, a group of PWAs from the United States sat down with our South African counterparts at a casual dinner party just outside of Cape Town.[1] It was a chilly night, but we were in the warm home of Zackie Achmat, a thirty-eight-year-old HIV-positive gay former anti-apartheid activist. Our host also chairs the Treatment Action Campaign (TAC), the three-year-old AIDS

1. This article was written a short time after the Thirteenth International AIDS Conference in Durban, South Africa. It records the efforts of the leading South African

organization that seized the world stage with a massive preconference protest march.

Achmat served delicious lamb and squash, and during the hours of boisterous conversation, we emptied several bottles of wine. At one point, we lapsed into silence, and Achmat seized the moment. He asked each of us Americans to pull out our HIV meds and show them to the assembled guests. A bit stunned, we reached into our pockets and laid our dozens of pills on the table. Bashfully, each of us explained the meds, their benefits and side effects. Achmat's gesture was brilliant, demonstrating the gross inequity among the PWAs in the room. Without polarizing his guests, he provoked a profound realization in the Americans: our South African dinner companions weren't angry at us—they simply want meds, too.

With just a few paid staffers but a large base of volunteers, TAC won its first victory on this front last November: the Medical Control Council (MCC), South Africa's drug regulators, granted a first-ever waiver allowing importation of a generic medication for the country's four million people with HIV. To accomplish this in a climate in which the government is ambivalent about acknowledging AIDS at all took international activist pressure. But it couldn't have happened without TAC's remarkable squad of HIV-positive South Africans.

The November success came after a nine-month campaign that included, at one point, the threat of U.S. sanctions and, at another, an offer by five pharmaceuticals to temporarily cut drug prices for southern Africa by eighty-five percent. TAC welcomed the discounts but condemned any

AIDS activist organization—the Treatment Action Campaign (TAC)—up until a few months after the conference. Since then there have been both many successes and setbacks. For a full history of TAC and updates on its campaigns see the group's web site: <http://tac.org.za>.

effort to keep the government from promoting importation or manufacture of even cheaper generic substitutes.

AIDS drugs are not prohibitively expensive to make. Manufacturers in India, Thailand, and Brazil have shown that most critical drugs, even antiretrovirals, can be produced at a cost that puts them within reach of the resource-poor world. Still, patent-holders inflate prices to deliver profits, and international trade laws block large-scale attempts to make and market the drugs at affordable prices. The World Trade Organization does allow countries facing a health emergency to authorize generic production of patented drugs. But there's no enforcement: countries that take this step still risk trade sanctions by powerful nations and well-funded lawsuits from international corporations.

Toward the end of the Durban conference, TAC called a press conference to announce its Defiance Campaign Against Patent Abuse and AIDS Profiteering: Starting with fluconazole, TAC would seek to make HIV- and opportunistic-infection (OI) meds accessible to all HIV-positive South Africans. Diflucan, Pfizer's patented fluconazole (used to treat thrush as well as a common and deadly OI, cryptococcal meningitis), retails for around seven dollars per pill; the South African government had been buying bulk from Pfizer for four dollars. Meanwhile, generic manufacturers in Thailand and India sell the drug for as low as twenty-nine cents.

Achmat announced that TAC would take legal action to seek a compulsory license that would allow South African generic production. He also held up a box of fluconazole and declared that TAC would break the law by importing a generic. Ingeniously, TAC had already set up a distribution network for the contraband drug, through doctors and nurses who had agreed to support the campaign. "As a doctor I have an ethical responsibility to my patients," Leon Geffen, M.D., told a local paper, "not to Pfizer or any other pharmaceutical."

Two months later, in mid-October, TAC activists did as promised: They defied South African patent law and imported 5,000 capsules of Biozole, the Thai version of fluconazole, and submitted a sample to the MCC for safety approval. At a press conference, Achmat was defiant: "TAC will stop breaking unjust trade laws once Pfizer has lowered the price to under four Rand [fifty cents] and its 'donation' is implemented with no restrictions." (In March 2000, Pfizer had offered to donate some Diflucan but set conditions so restrictive the offer has yet to be implemented.) The MCC responded by charging Achmat with illegal importation of drugs.

On October 20, flanked by political and religious leaders, Zackie Achmat surrendered himself to police in Cape Town. "Comrades," he said, "it is a very sad moment when we know medications can save our lives, but we have to break the law to get access to them." The activist who had been beaten by the police in the late seventies while incarcerated for his anti-apartheid efforts was again facing interrogation by white police officers. This time, Achmat says, the officers were polite. One even offered words of support. But while policing may have changed since the anti-apartheid movement, Achmat says that the lessons of that long struggle against racism must now be applied to AIDS. In particular, he mentions the value of winning real victories rather than simply making noise. By succeeding with fluconazole, he says, the group has something to build on.

Achmat says another lesson of the anti-apartheid movement is the need to build a strong political culture—one that supports and protects people with HIV. Only last August, a young teacher, Mpho Motloung, twenty-five, of Soweto was killed by her husband in a murder-suicide. On her body was a note with the words "HIV Positive AIDS." Struggling to understand the crime, Achmat sent an e-mail to international supporters blaming the South African government. He wrote: "Everywhere we go, we hear: 'HIV/AIDS is a death sentence' or, worse, 'There is no cure: Education and prevention is the only protection.' From these primitive messages, people learn fear, hopelessness, loneliness and anger. . . . Government messages fail to tell the millions of people with HIV that it is possible to live fully and productively for many years."

To combat this despair with hope and solidarity, TAC has cultivated a new generation of HIV-positive activists, such as Promise Mthembu, twenty-six. "Being open and public about my HIV status is helping me to take out all of my frustrations and anger," she says. "I feel that I'm helping other people with HIV who cannot speak out." Mthembu, a former HIV counselor, quickly emerged as a TAC leader and now coordinates the group's Kwazulu-Natal office and serves on TAC's executive committee. But her treatment options are typical of all but South Africa's wealthiest: a handful of antibiotics and other OI meds, but no antiretrovirals at all. Although testing facilities are available, Mthembu stopped getting her CD4 counts because, she says, they always drop. "I don't see the need for me to go for testing because the numbers are not going to improve anyway." Mthembu has never had her nine-year-old daughter tested for HIV. Without access to treatments, Mthembu says, knowing her child's HIV status would be intolerable.

While approximately 5,000 HIV-positive babies are born in South Africa each month, a government pilot program, which makes nevirapine available to lower the risk of mother-to-child transmission, covers a mere five percent of pregnant women. Mthembu coordinates another of TAC's fights: to force the government to make these meds universally available to positive mothers-to-be.

At the National AIDS Treatment Advocates Forum in Dallas last November, Achmat and Mthembu each spoke at the opening plenary, calling on PWAs in the United States to support the Defiance Campaign by pushing U.S.-based pharmaceuticals to donate AIDS drugs to poor nations and pressuring our government to ease trade restrictions that prevent generic importing (even more urgent with a Bush presidency). After Mthembu

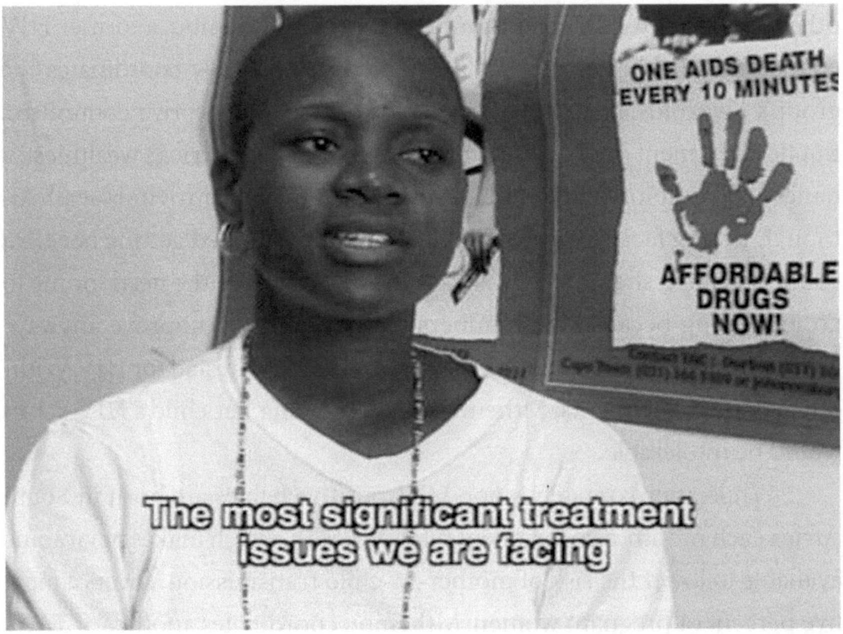

Figure 10.2 Promise Mthembu. From Gregg Bordowitz, *Habit*, 2001.

spoke, advocates from around the United States took her aside to persuade her to take care of her own health while she fights for treatment access for others. Mthembu decided to get her CD4 count upon returning home, and then to pursue getting Bactrim (a pneumonia prophylaxis the government has pledged to provide) and whatever else is easily available to her in South Africa. After that, she says, she'll consider seeking help from people in the United States to obtain whatever additional drugs she may need.

Supporters have offered to purchase HAART[2] meds for Achmat outright, but he's publically declared that he will not take any drugs unless they are available to everyone in South Africa. Since his government does provide a handful of medications to treat opportunistic infections, Achmat will, if necessary, take these meds. But he told me, "I have decided not to take antiretrovirals because I don't want to live in a world that devalues the lives of poor people simply because they are poor. I could never look those people in the eye, and I couldn't lead them, if I was taking my medicines while they were going to die."

Achmat's pledge, in the courageous tradition of Ghandi's hunger strikes and Nelson Mandela's refusal to renounce armed struggle to get out of prison, is a display of the kind of moral leadership that could turn around the AIDS epidemic.[3] In three short years, TAC has not only pushed

2. HAART is an acronym for "highly active antiretroviral therapy."

3. Zackie Achmat recently announced that he will begin taking antiretroviral therapy. "I'm not going to die because they want us to die." The leadership of TAC recognized that his death would be devastating for the movement. Nathan Geffen, a spokesperson for TAC was quoted by the Associated Press, "We need Zackie to live through this and not become a victim of the government's denialism and arrogance." See "Africa: AIDS activist ends drug strike," accessed from planetout.com, August 5, 2003.

The South African government has finally agreed to provide treatment to people with AIDS. See "South Africa Addresses AIDS," *New York Times,* Editorial, August 18, 2003.

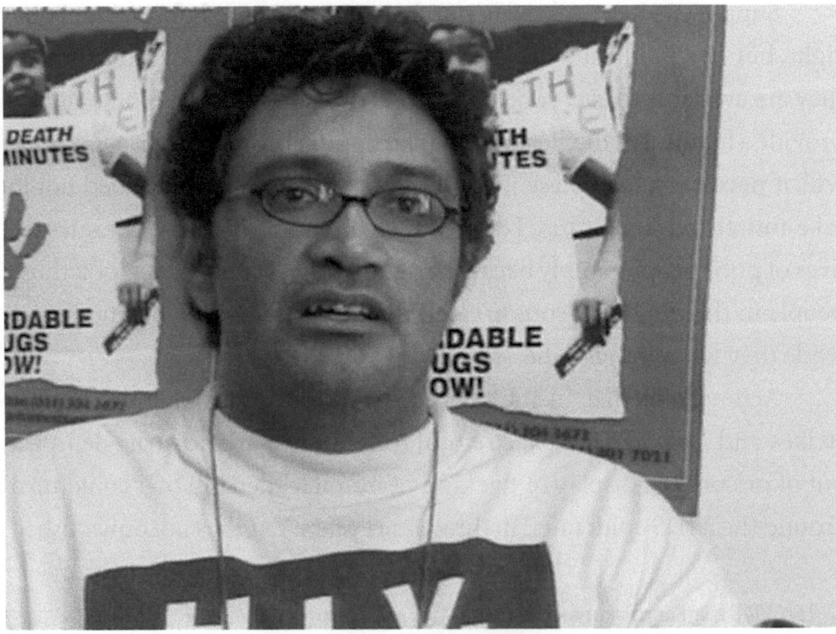

Figure 10.3 Zackie Achmat. From Gregg Bordowitz, *Habit*, 2001.

the South African government to expand HIV drug access, it has helped establish an activist network among poor nations producing, procuring, and distributing quality medicines despite trade restrictions and pharmaceutical industry pressure.

With each bit of progress comes resistance. In January, South African TV star Morne Visser arrived at Cape Town International Airport with a now legal shipment of Thai fluconazole. As he entered the arrivals hall, Visser was lifted into the air by more than one hundred delighted TAC supporters. Then, in early March, oral arguments began in the Pretoria High Court as some forty pharmaceutical firms sued the South African government over a 1997 law allowing importation or production of generic drugs.

For now, Achmat remains relatively healthy, and for that he credits his involvement with TAC: "It's the activism that pushed my CD4 counts up. It's the fact that I have so many more friends now—people with and without HIV—because they realize that we are doing something together and we can win. Not because of the stand I've taken, but because TAC is giving them hope."

The Effort to Survive AIDS Considered from the Point of View of a Race-Car Driver

11

Originally published as "The Effort to Survive AIDS Considered from the Point of View of a Race-Car Driver," in Gregg Bordowitz, *Drive: The AIDS Crisis Is Still Beginning* (Chicago: Whitewalls, 2002), pp. 72–75. Minor revisions have been made for consistency.

THIS TEXT AND ITS TITLE WERE INSPIRED *by J. G. Ballard, "The Assassination of John Fitzgerald Kennedy Considered as a Downhill Motor Race,"* The Atrocity Exhibition *(San Francisco, Calif.: RE/Search Publications, 1990), pp. 108–109. Ballard's text refers to Alfred Jarry's "The Crucifixion Considered as an Uphill Bicycle Race."*

Chapter 11
From the POV of a Race-Car Driver

All racers need more horsepower. Unfortunately, there aren't many things that entry-level racers can do to get more power out of their engines without spending thousands and thousands of dollars. To get the horsepower you need, you might have to break the rules, your budget, or both. 215

Bear in mind that the driving conditions imagined by the original engine manufacturer differ wildly from those you subject your engine to

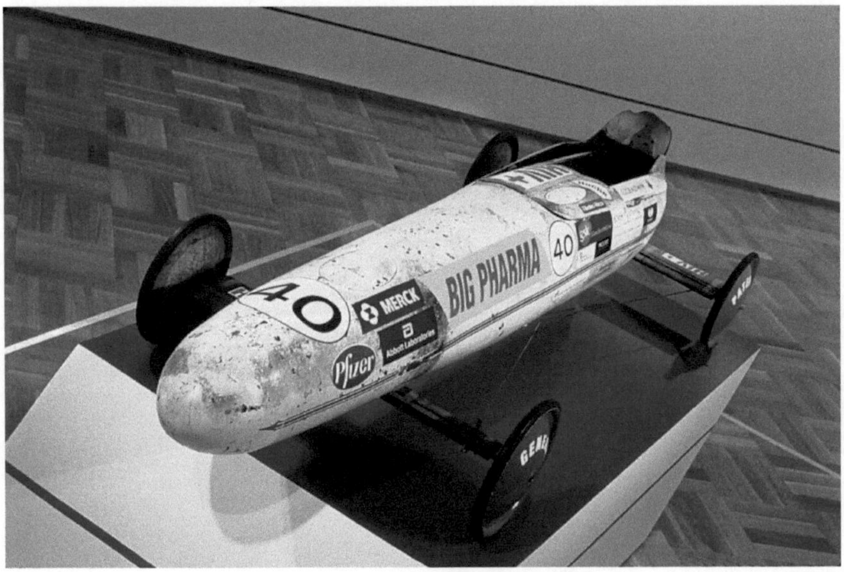

Figure 11.1 Gregg Bordowitz, *Drive,* 2002. Courtesy of the Museum of Contemporary Art, Chicago. Exhibition photography © 2002 Museum of Contemporary Art, Chicago. Photo by James Isberner.

while racing. Fuel requirements, emission standards, and normal life-span projections determine standard tune-up recommendations. There are some things you can do simply by returning to the manufacturer's settings, assuming you have a stock engine that remains in basically sound condition. Begin by following basic rules of car ownership, such as using the right fuel and getting regular tune-ups and oil changes. Rookie racers consider these hints: rejet your carburetor to make it significantly richer. Increase the amount of air that your engine pumps by blocking off the heat riser in your intake manifold. Always use fresh plugs.

Of course, there are things to consider other than the engine. (If your engine is making strange sounds or is vibrating badly, it is probably a waste of time and money to try to improve its performance with a simple tweak here and there. You need help.) An important factor is the final drive ratio. Look at your numbers just before you lift going into the turns. If they're not consistent with your engine's safe operating speed, you need more gear. Determining what kind of gear you need requires a fair amount of diagnostic work.

Loads. Back off the factory-recommended measures and establish a new baseline with repeat testing. The CD4 count, the CD4–CD8 ratio, and, most important, the viral load are all significant indicators of how the system is running. These tests are expensive and most racers need sponsorship to get them. Many who can't find the big money sponsors refuse to consider taking these vital tests, since the information you'll get will probably just slow you down if you don't have the gear to improve your numbers.

Transmissions. Getting infected with the racing bug remains a central concern for everyone, on and off the field. The race gets increasingly difficult to run with more and more cars on the track. The less infections, the better, obviously. The growing number of racers in spite of years of safety campaigns is a testament to the limits of driver education. (Most campaigns have been flawed, underfunded, and compromised.)

Even seasoned drivers should be concerned with transmission, both to protect others' safety and their own. Exposure to all kinds of elements can diminish your drive. The need for speed is a common desire. Most of us balance our safety with our desires, each determining our own behaviors according to what makes life worthwhile.

Switching your gear repeatedly can be hazardous. Carrying the latest gear will often keep you running at a decent speed, but the best gear wears out fast, requiring changes mid-race. Use of gear combinations often brings a mixed bag of unforeseen and unintended snags and snarls that foul up weight, speed, emissions, fuel intake, appearance, and any number of other things important to the racer. It's best to keep yourself out of the race. Though it may look exciting from the stands, it's terrifying on the track.

I've been driving a long time and I'd be lying if I said that I am not as concerned with winning as I am with finishing. (The likelihood of either seems to be receding into the distance.) Still, I am lucky. By the graces of chance, I've got sponsors, an excellent crew chief, and a well-organized team. There are plenty out there who, for reasons of greed mostly, can't find a sponsor. Imagine being a driver without a ride. That's hell. Every racer deserves a ride. Forget the track, forget the sport, and forget the win—if you need to run you've been cursed with something beyond your control. Call it bad luck, call it whatever you want, you didn't ask for it, and even if you feel that you did, as many of us do, no one deserves it.

Multitudes. Racing is among the fastest-growing sports. All around the world, there are drivers looking for sponsors and a team that will lead them to glory. Many places in the world offer neither a decent track to run on, nor the proper equipment to drive. The latest gear is available only in a few shops around the world.

That's not going to stop drivers from racing. Every driver needs to drive. Without drivers, there is no sport. If the drivers get organized, we

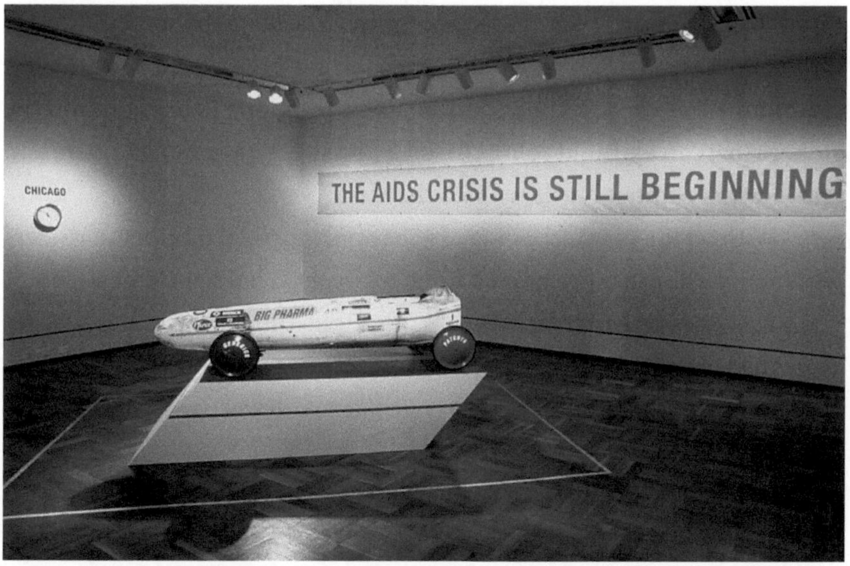

Figure 11.2 Gregg Bordowitz, *Drive,* 2002. Courtesy of the Museum of Contemporary Art, Chicago. Exhibition photography © 2002 Museum of Contemporary Art, Chicago. Photo by James Isberner.

can make the rules. We're more powerful than the sponsors. They depend on us for their livelihood. Collectively, we're more powerful than the global governing bodies that make the rules of the sport. Their leadership isn't democratically selected. That's the problem. Ideally, they should hold office to serve the sport, not the sponsors.

Some say the great diversity among races is a big problem for the sport. This is not a problem for drivers. Yes, the tracks and the vehicles differ from situation to situation. Licensed or outlaw, it's all racing to us: stock cars, Formula 1, sprint cars, carts and funny cars. Even the soapbox derby. It's all about the drive. The two most important problems for the drivers are: How do we capture the common purpose among drivers around the globe? How can we build solidarity on a massive scale among drivers and fans? Racers without borders, that's the ideal.

With all the new technology in the sport, a small number of drivers with major sponsors are having longer careers. That's good news, but it often eclipses the harsh fact that all of us, old-timers and rookies alike, share the same fate. Today, a fatal crash is the inevitable end of every driver. Even those of us with access to every privilege a driver can imagine fall to the sport.

So, what does it mean to win? As it is now, we're pitted against each other, competing for the sponsors' interests. Yet, we don't race for the sponsors. All drivers race out of necessity, certainly not by choice, and most of the drivers in the world can't find sponsorship. Inequity in racing ruins integrity in the sport. Sure, there are trophies and prize money, merchandise and commercial endorsements. These rewards are fleeting and illusory. You're always facing the next car race. It's always a hellish return to the same. We drive, some of us get famous, sponsors get rich, and spectators continue to fill the stands.

My Postmodernism

12

Originally published as "My Postmodernism," *Artforum* 41, no. 7 (March 2003): 226–229, 273–274. Minor revisions have been made for consistency.

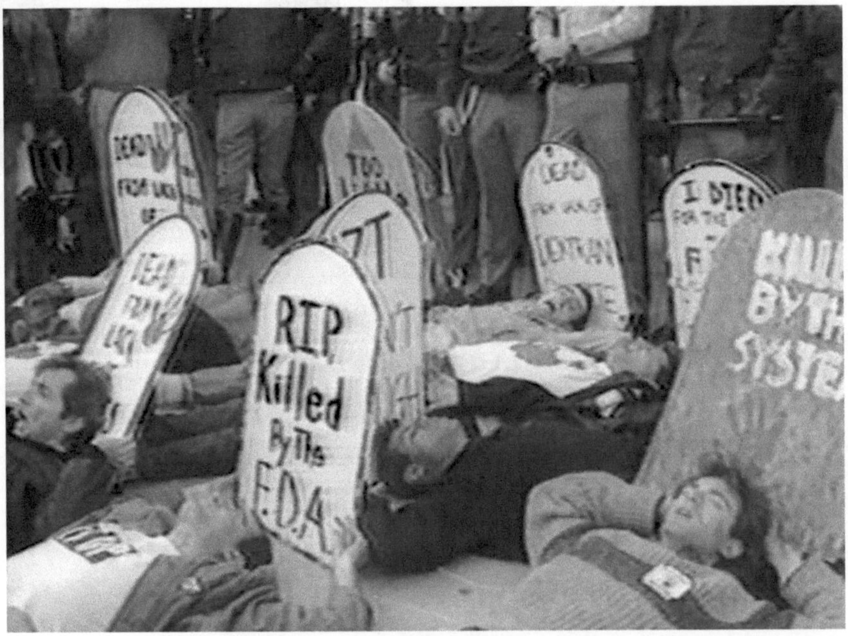

Figure 12.1 Gregg Bordowitz, *Fast Trip, Long Drop*, 1993.

Art does have the power to save lives, and it is this very power that must be recognized, fostered, and supported in every way possible. —*Douglas Crimp, introduction to* AIDS: Cultural Analysis/Cultural Activism

Chapter 12
My Postmodernism

[**Identity**]

When Ronald Reagan was elected president, I was sixteen years old, living in Coram, Long Island. A smart faggy teen, I spent every possible minute drawing and painting in the art rooms of Longwood High School. I loved Jackson Pollock *and* Andy Warhol. I listened to an eclectic mix of music, including

Miles Davis, James Brown, and the Ramones. It was my girlfriend Michelle who introduced me to punk culture. She taught me everything I needed to know—where to get the music, where to shop for jewelry (any pet store), and how to cut my own hair without a mirror. Well, almost everything. My crush on one of Longwood's art teachers led to the other defining friendship of my high school years. Mr. ______ instructed me in the ways of the gay world, even taking me into the city and showing me the leather shops and bookstores of the West Village. I always knew that the minute I turned eighteen I would move to Manhattan, which seemed as far away and glamorous as Hollywood. After graduating, I followed Michelle to the School of Visual Arts.

On arrival in Manhattan, I made friends with others new to the city. During the day we studied art and visited museums. At night we explored bars. I recall one late night at the Pyramid Club on Avenue A in the East Village. The house was packed, and there was a long list of entertainers. A tall slender blond boy dressed in metallic space gear tapped out a scale repeatedly on a toy electronic organ. In a trancelike state, he chanted, "Take what you can get and call it love."

I spent the next four years in and out of love with many men and women. I formed important and enduring friendships with artists like Mark Dion, Jason Simon, and Andrea Fraser. In 1986, Andrea and I lived together, on Fourth Street between A and B. The East Village was then host to a hodgepodge of cultures—punk, bohemian, queer, and druggie. No one I knew referred to himself as gay. That identity was reserved for clones—older homosexual men who wore mustaches and dressed alike in tight jeans and nylon bomber jackets, or in leather. I rejected this style as a kind of conformity. I was free of labels.

None of my friends knew much about AIDS in 1986. I was still living in a mostly straight-identified scene, and AIDS was a remote concern. But then the reports about the AIDS crisis that began to dominate the news captured my attention, probably because I realized that I could have become exposed to HIV from sex with any number of men—some friends, some acquaintances, some strangers. Even among my few homosexual friends there was much confusion, misinformation, and denial when it came to safe sex. The public sex culture of gay life that had achieved visibility and legitimacy through the sexual revolution was being driven underground by homophobia. In the mid-eighties, mandatory testing and quarantine were discussed at very high levels of the Reagan administration.

Underlying all this confusion was the fear that one could test positive and die a horrible death very quickly. This fear, magnified by all the attention AIDS was getting in the news, drove me to seek advice and information. The only hospitable place to go was the Lesbian and Gay Community Services Center on Thirteenth Street, between Seventh and Eighth Avenues. I became acquainted with the center through my work protesting the 1986 Supreme Court ruling (*Bowers v. Hardwick*) that upheld state sodomy laws. *Hardwick* reinvigorated the gay-rights movement, as hundreds of people turned out for marches and demonstrations in New York. I videotaped these protests—my fledgling efforts as an activist documentarian. This activity led me to form more friendships with gay men and lesbians.

The community center was a somewhat run-down old building four or five stories high. In the warm weather, there were always people hanging out outside, smoking and talking. The inside badly needed a paint job. The stained surfaces of the walls were peeling. It was a labyrinth of different-size rooms, rooms within rooms, a couple of staircases. For me, it all added to the allure of the place. Clearly the imperative to provide shelter for gay men and lesbians, to foster an affirming culture, was more important than appearances. A sign on an easel just inside the main entrance listed dozens of meetings, consciousness-raising and discussion groups of all kinds concerning communities within the larger community—leather men, men of all colors together, the Salsa Soul Sisters, Alcoholics Anonymous, poetry readings, and so on.

The Community Health Project was on the second floor. Climbing the red staircase put me in mind of fire drills at my elementary school. At the CHP, I was given a free examination and much-needed sex education, all dispensed without judgment. The health care workers on staff didn't know me, but I could tell they'd helped many people like me. The experience was profound, a revelation: community is the space claimed and defended by people who need one another. On the steps of the center that day, I decided to become a citizen of the gay community, and I vowed to make a contribution to it.

[**Ideology**]

In 1985, I attended the Whitney Museum of American Art's Independent Study Program, a university-level program for artists, curators, and critics who draw on critical theory in their work. The curriculum consisted of weekly reading seminars and presentations given by a prestigious list of visiting faculty. The weekly reading group was central to my experience of the ISP. Under the stewardship of the program's much-loved director, Ron Clark, it was organized in a way that reminded me of Hebrew school, a very pleasant association. Ron always led the group, sitting at the head of the long table. The students sat around it with their texts open, marked with notes. Ron assigned readings by Jacques Derrida, Michel Foucault, Luce Irigaray, Laura Mulvey, Jacques Lacan, and Louis Althusser. Reading Althusser opened our eyes to the notion that ideology is a worldview constructed through language itself, the very medium of social life. We speak language and it speaks us. Ideology works from the core of identity, mediating our relations with others.

Change is not simply a matter of developing better ideas and convincing others of their validity. Radical change is a matter of altering the entire culture's view of reality. All around me, people were getting sick, living in fear of dying, losing others. The government didn't care. President Reagan refused to acknowledge the crisis publicly, and televangelist Jerry Falwell seemed almost gleeful in pronouncing AIDS to be an example of God's wrath against homosexuals. In a period marked by increasing homophobia, racism, xenophobia, poverty, and homelessness—all exacerbated by Republican social policy—a revolutionary change of consciousness was necessary.

Craig Owens (1950–1990) taught at the Whitney program. A trained art historian whose work would evolve into deconstructionist criticism and theory, Craig was a gay man who identified as a male feminist. By the mid-eighties, he was struggling to apply feminist theory and psychoanalysis to homosexuality. He hesitated. It was a big decision. Discussing homosexuality entailed coming out publicly in the professional world, and that unavoidably led one into identity politics. There were risks for intellectuals then, as there are now. You risk having all your work reduced and dismissed. More than that, there were strong arguments against coming out. Foucault, for instance, suspected the coming-out narrative as a means of incorporation into a juridical-medical-disciplinary regime. Eventually, though, Foucault came out. And Craig wrote a piece titled "Outlaws: Gay Men in Feminism" (1987).

[Illusion]

Craig's Upper West Side apartment was cluttered with stacks of books because there was no more space on his bookshelves. In this environment, I was first introduced to Schönberg's opera *Moses und Aron*. Craig slowly took the LP out of its sleeve, careful not to get any fingerprints on the vinyl. I sat still, keeping my excitement a secret. The needle dropped, and after a few revolutions the strangest sounds emanated from the speakers. I had never heard music like that before.

Schönberg's libretto retells the Old Testament story of the golden calf as a parable for an aesthetic debate concerning Truth versus Appearance—a debate central to the work of Theodor Adorno and the Frankfurt School. Suspicions concerning the seductive nature of images, the disproportionate role of the modern media in shaping public opinion, and the exploitation of the power of images by Nazi propagandists all combined to amplify the relevance of the biblical debate, which haunted postwar discussions of art and culture. Abstract expressionism came to eschew representation altogether in its quest for transcendental Truth, while the conceptual artists of the sixties and seventies shared the Hebraic preference for word over image. In the early eighties the terms of the debate were turned upside down.

In New York, a group of artists associated with Metro Pictures worked in a conceptual vein but chose to flaunt the very images that their predecessors had so rigorously rejected. Indeed, they made the Golden Calf (i.e., products of the culture industry) the very subject of their work. But artists like Barbara Kruger, Richard Prince, and Sherrie Levine didn't produce ostentatious images; in brazen acts of *détournement* they appropriated them, turning them against the very culture industry that had put them into circulation in the first place. Kruger went so far as to combine word and image, acutely aware that, in this age of advertising, the word *is* an image (think logo). The appropriationists weren't preoccupied with specific pictures so much as with critiquing—or deconstructing, as one might have said at the time—an entire regime of image production. These were among the artists Craig Owens championed.

[Immunity]

My nagging suspicions about my HIV status proved correct. In 1988, accompanied by my friend Rebecca, I received a positive result through an anonymous testing program at a clinic on Ninth Avenue around Twenty-eighth Street. Outside the clinic's entrance was a statue commemorating the naval war dead. A solitary stone figure of a sailor stood erect, stoically looking off into the space above your head. Exiting the clinic, I paused in front of the statue and remembered the first line of Jean Genet's novel *Querelle:* "The notion of murder often brings to mind the notion of sea and sailors."

[Impulse]

When I tested HIV positive the gay community had an ethos: everyone with AIDS was innocent. No blame could be attached to a seropositive status. All infections were assumed to be caused by ignorance. I was first introduced to safer-sex education in 1985, perhaps even earlier, and still I didn't practice safer sex consistently until I tested positive. The role of the unconscious cannot be underestimated when it comes to the difficulties of practicing safer sex. The idea that you can't do what you strongly desire, for the rest of your life, is profoundly painful.

Today, responses to recent seroconversions are ambivalent, sometimes even hostile. For those of us who have lost scores of people, the thought of another prolonged illness and death is intolerable. But there's an objectionable kind of moralism that's crept into the gay community. People who seroconvert now are viewed with suspicion. A person can be made to feel that he has perpetrated violence against himself. If we give in to this kind of thinking, we neglect to acknowledge the violence perpetrated against our sexual lives by the epidemic itself, and the difficulties of remaining HIV-negative.

[Incontinence]

I worked at Gay Men's Health Crisis from 1988 to 1993. At GMHC, my friend Jean Carlomusto and I coproduced a weekly public-access cable show called *Living with AIDS.* The program was made by and for people with AIDS and those who loved and supported them. Jean and I thought of ourselves as part of a counterculture making work for an audience of people excluded by the television industry, which presumed its audience to be uninfected and unaffected. I remember when a colleague who was suffering tremendously from wasting showed up to work at GMHC wearing brand-new white sweatpants. He had a huge brown diarrhea stain on his ass. He was embarrassed and ashamed that he had lost control of his bowels on the subway. Loss of control is perhaps the most frightening aspect of AIDS—loss of control over your functions, over your weight, over your health in general. Illness was visible everywhere in New York in the eighties. Tormented by ubiquitous signs of distress, my generation of activist artists worked to affirm life.

[Inertia]

I was very busy in the late eighties. In 1987, a small group of gay men and their concerned friends founded ACT UP, to do what nonprofit service organizations like GMHC could not possibly do: take militant direct action

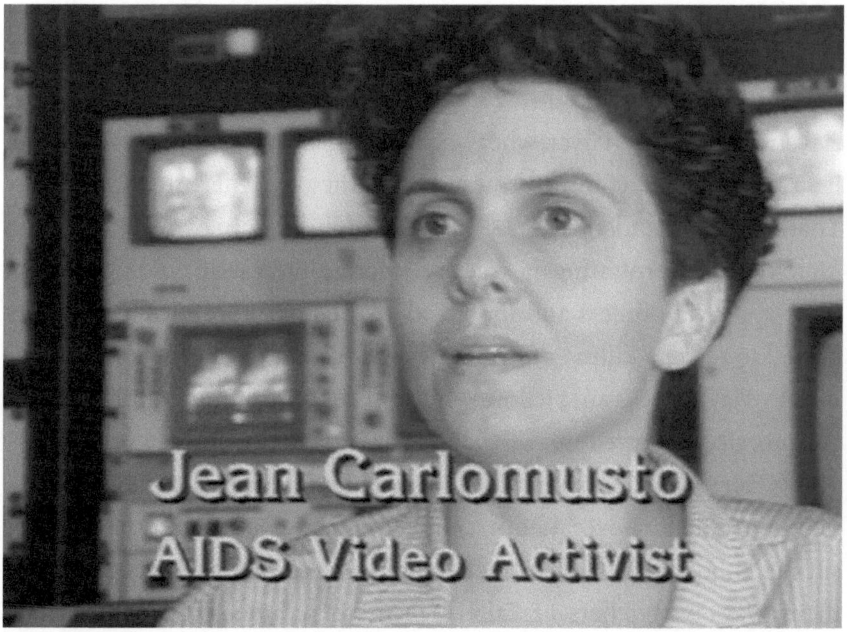

Figure 12.2 Jean Carlomusto. From Gregg Bordowitz, *Fast Trip, Long Drop*, 1993.

against the government. But even before ACT UP was officially formed, there were signs of an emerging AIDS-activist movement. A provocative poster appeared around town—a pink triangle on a black background bearing the words SILENCE = DEATH. A small group of gay men (who would later form Gran Fury with other activists) designed this poster, and they had copies "sniped" at their own expense. The design was given to ACT UP to use at an early action, and "SILENCE = DEATH" was adopted as the organization's slogan.

At that time, I looked to the city's walls for direction. I recall exiting the Christopher Street subway station when a small eight-and-a-half-by-eleven-inch Xeroxed flyer, wheat-pasted to the wall, caught my attention. It advertised an upcoming protest. I knew then and there that I would go. That's how I attended ACT UP's first demonstration, on Wall Street on March 24, 1987, protesting the role of corporate interests in guiding the FDA drug-approval process and the greed of the pharmaceutical companies poised to make a killing off the drugs we desperately needed. Accompanied by David Meieran, a fellow Whitney Program alumnus and a creative collaborator, I showed up with a video camera to document the event.

Over 250 people gathered in front of Trinity Church at 7:00 A.M. We tied up traffic for several hours, and seventeen people were arrested for sitting in the middle of the street and refusing to get up. The cops carried them away on stretchers. I recall two protesters connected by a thick chain wrapped around their torsos—a young white man wearing a beret and a gray-haired woman wrapped in a heavy wool overcoat. The morning was cold and gray. Flashes of light from the cameras of many news photographers added to the stormy atmosphere. TV news crews jostled each other to get the better shots. (With a small consumer VHS camera, I had yet to learn how to hold my own among the burly cameramen with bigger rigs.)

Most of the protesters were packed together on the sidewalk behind police barricades. The cops were prepared for the event and treated the protesters gently. (If I remember correctly, the terms of the nonviolent protest were negotiated with the police before the event. Experienced activists had been doing that for years. Later, the practice would be challenged by a new generation of organizers.) A tall African-American man with a megaphone—I think his name was Charles—led the crowd in chants: "More AIDS drugs are what we need. All we get is profit and greed." An effigy of the FDA commissioner, Frank Young, was strung up by its neck from a street lamp. Passersby moved quickly away from the scene. We called after them, "You can get it too."

As an artist, I felt that I had a unique contribution to make to AIDS activism: I could use my skills as a manipulator of images to document the movement from the point of view of activists. I was biased. I was partisan. And I was not alone. A generation of artists joined the cause and freely gave their time and expertise to produce a vibrant culture in the interests of people with AIDS. The videos I worked on collectively with so many others, too numerous to mention here, were skilled constructions intended to incite people to action.

Looking back now at that intensely prolific period, when I never went anywhere without a camera, I can see myself: panicky, hyper, moody, arrogant, and filled with love for my fellow activists. I was also depressed, weighed down by self-criticism, anxious, and afraid. I rarely, if ever, showed up to work at GMHC on time. I slept little at night in those years. When I did finally fall asleep, very early in the morning, I was often too tired to get to work on time. Too terrified to face the day. It's a mystery to me how I was eventually able to get out of bed and work tirelessly all day and into the night.

[Inheritance]

I had wanted to be an artist ever since I was a child. I never wanted to be anything else. Though I feared that the art I was making as an activist strayed from my initial goal, I never let go of my absorption with aesthetic concerns. Yvonne Rainer was my greatest influence. Her kaleidoscopic films like *Journeys from Berlin/1971* (1980) and *The Man Who Envied Women* (1985) drew directly from the theoretical debates of the day. Those works showed me how to respond to the historical present. Robert Smithson was important to me too. For Smithson, writing was *the* model for art production, and he made language itself the ground of his practice (as Craig Owens had argued in his 1979 essay "Earthwords"). From 1983 to 1985, I was Joseph Kosuth's studio assistant. He taught me that the meaning of a work of art did not emanate from the work itself but rather from the ways it was discussed. There were many other influences: Soviet cinema, the Situationists, Daniel Buren, Dee Dee Halleck, Paper Tiger Television, and Martha Rosler.

[Intervention]

My friend Charles Barber, a poet, refused to accept his disease as a terrible death to be suffered in silence. He used wordplay to fiercely reject the destiny and social isolation enforced by the use of the acronym AIDS and the stigma attached to it. At an early ACT UP rally, he stood in the rain, reading to a crowd from a soggy piece of paper. Playing on the acronym's potential, Charles defined AIDS as Acquired Internal Doubt of Self.

ACT UP's greatest strength was its primary commitment to the concerns of people with AIDS. People came to ACT UP because they were sick

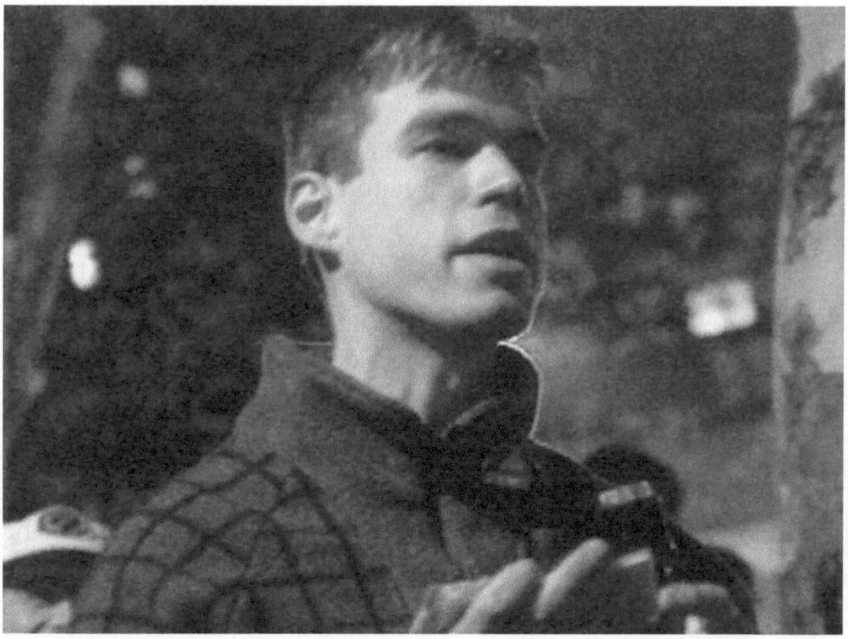

Figure 12.3 Charles Barber. From Gregg Bordowitz, *Fast Trip, Long Drop,* 1993.

or because their lovers were sick. Their friends had AIDS. Their father or their brother was dying. Few people in the group were activists before AIDS. Everyone involved was willing to use just about any means possible to end AIDS. This commitment superseded traditional left politics and the sectarianism that has so often paralyzed progressive efforts.

ACT UP didn't have a policy on media. Some people used their connections in show business, advertising, or the art world to publicize our cause. Other activists, like me, labored to establish a vibrant alternative media. In established left politics these two tactics—using the media or creating your own—were considered mutually exclusive. In ACT UP, if we thought something would help people with AIDS, we did it. And no theoretical antinomy between "dominant culture" and "counterculture" would stop us.

ACT UP at its height, between 1988 and 1991, was an extraordinarily diverse group. Of course, there were tensions between lesbians and gay men, between people of color and white people, between the HIV-positive and the HIV-negative, and so on. Nevertheless, my experience with ACT UP was probably the closest I will ever come to working in a true coalition. We embraced our contradictions. We were serious, angry, defiant, and proud. We were silly, theatrical, campy, and irreverent. We were sexy. The regular Monday night general meeting was the hottest place to be in New York. Over five hundred people crammed into the first floor of the Lesbian and Gay Community Services Center. You had to touch a hundred bodies to cross the room. It was a great place to cruise.

Early on ACT UP adopted Robert's Rules of Order for its procedures. Two facilitators elected by the group ran the general Monday night meetings. Issues were discussed within agreed-on time periods. Decisions were voted on and carried by a majority. We were extremely efficient and would complete an enormous amount of business in a single night. Meetings lasted three, sometimes four hours. Much business was conducted on the periphery of the general meeting, at the edges of the crowd, or in side rooms. ACT UP comprised a number of small committees—action, media, treatment, and data, and so on—which met at varying times, so there was a different committee meeting every night of the week. There was also a caucus organized by people of color. All these groups reported to the general meeting, and their presentations were at times boring, at others exhilarating. Our camp sensibility made for hilarious moments. And we often cried. The names of the recently deceased were announced at every meeting. After the meetings, we continued our conversations in bars and restaurants all over the Village.

The most significant political action that I helped organize was the nonviolent takeover of the FDA headquarters in Rockville, Maryland, on October 11, 1988. ACT UP groups from around the country converged on the bureaucracy's headquarters. Around fifteen hundred people participated. Many were organized into smaller cells, called "affinity groups." The affinity groups functioned autonomously, each determining its own focus, schedule, and approach. One affinity group called itself Surrender Dorothy (after *The Wizard of Oz*). I recall another group dressed in white lab coats, their outfits and hands smeared with red paint, chanting, "The FDA has blood on its hands, and we're seeing red." Some activists scaled the walls, using ladders to climb onto window ledges and paste signs on the windows. Others commandeered the flagpoles outside the building, hoisting huge banners to replace the Stars and Stripes. A couple of windows were broken. A few people wrestled with the cops, unsuccessfully trying to force their way through a side entrance. The police for the most part focused on preventing demonstrators from entering the premises. Surprisingly few arrests were made—176. With separate groups roaming around the headquarters doing their own actions, at times staggered throughout the day, we were able to shut the building down. We chanted, "Seize control," over and over as we advanced on the building. Our intention was to take over the sluggish agency and run it in the interests of people with AIDS.

Obviously we didn't permanently take over the FDA, but our actions led to significant reforms. Most important, the number of people with HIV who could get access to experimental drugs was greatly increased through expanded trials. The FDA and other government organizations started to listen to us. Members of ACT UP were consulted and invited to attend meetings. The organizers realized the FDA takeover was a watershed moment when we watched the national news in a motel room immediately following the action. It was covered on virtually every news program. Peter Staley, an HIV-positive ACT UP activist, faced Pat Buchanan on *Crossfire.* We had successfully wrested the public discussion on AIDS out of the hands of the right wing.

At first, AIDS activism had been a defensive battle. We were trying to keep ourselves from being mandatorily tested, even quarantined. Like warriors in a martial-arts film, we turned the opponent's weight against him. Faced with discrimination, we organized. In 1988 a decisive turn was made. The action against the FDA was a tour de force of nonviolent civil disobedience. After that, AIDS activism went on the offensive. We demanded that people with AIDS be involved at every level of decision making concerning all medical research and treatment for our disease. And we changed everything. We changed the way research is conducted. We changed the way patients are viewed. We changed the way drugs are developed, tested, and sold. Our uncompromising demand to give people with AIDS power over decisions affecting their lives is *the* lasting historical contribution of ACT UP.

AIDS activism can now be viewed historically, but it would be criminal to imply that the crisis is over. According to UNAIDS, forty-two million people are infected with HIV worldwide. Only a small fraction of people with HIV can get access to treatment and care. Without a coordinated, well-financed response, the epidemic will kill unimaginable numbers by the decade's end. The AIDS crisis is still beginning.

13

More Operative Assumptions

I WROTE THIS TEXT FOR JAMES MEYER. *James likes the earlier essay "Operative Assumptions." This new text picks up where that essay left off. I borrowed from various texts to write portions of this essay: "Art of Living: James Meyer talks with Gregg Bordowitz,"* Artforum *33, no. 10 (summer 1995): 89–90, 128; "Fast Trip, Long View: Talking to Gregg Bordowitz," interview with Robert Atkins,* Artery: The AIDS-Arts Journal *(summer 2000), <www.artistswithaids.org/artery/index1.html>; Richard Morrison, "Force of Habit," unpublished interview with Gregg Bordowitz, 2003; Douglas Crimp and Gregg Bordowitz, "A Noun and a Verb," in Gregg Bordowitz,* Drive: The AIDS Crisis Is Still Beginning *(Chicago: whitewalls, 2002), pp. 29–38.*

Utter vanity—said Koheleth—
Utter vanity! All is vanity!
What real value is there for a man
In all the gains he makes beneath the sun?[1]

Chapter 13
More Operative Assumptions

[Figure A.]

The presence of a camera in any situation mobilizes an order of image production. This order is a system in disequilibrium; like a whirlpool, its substance swirls around a hollow vortex. The camera occupies the center. Time is the one element that unifies the chaotic structure. The term

1. Ecclesiastes 1:1–1:3.

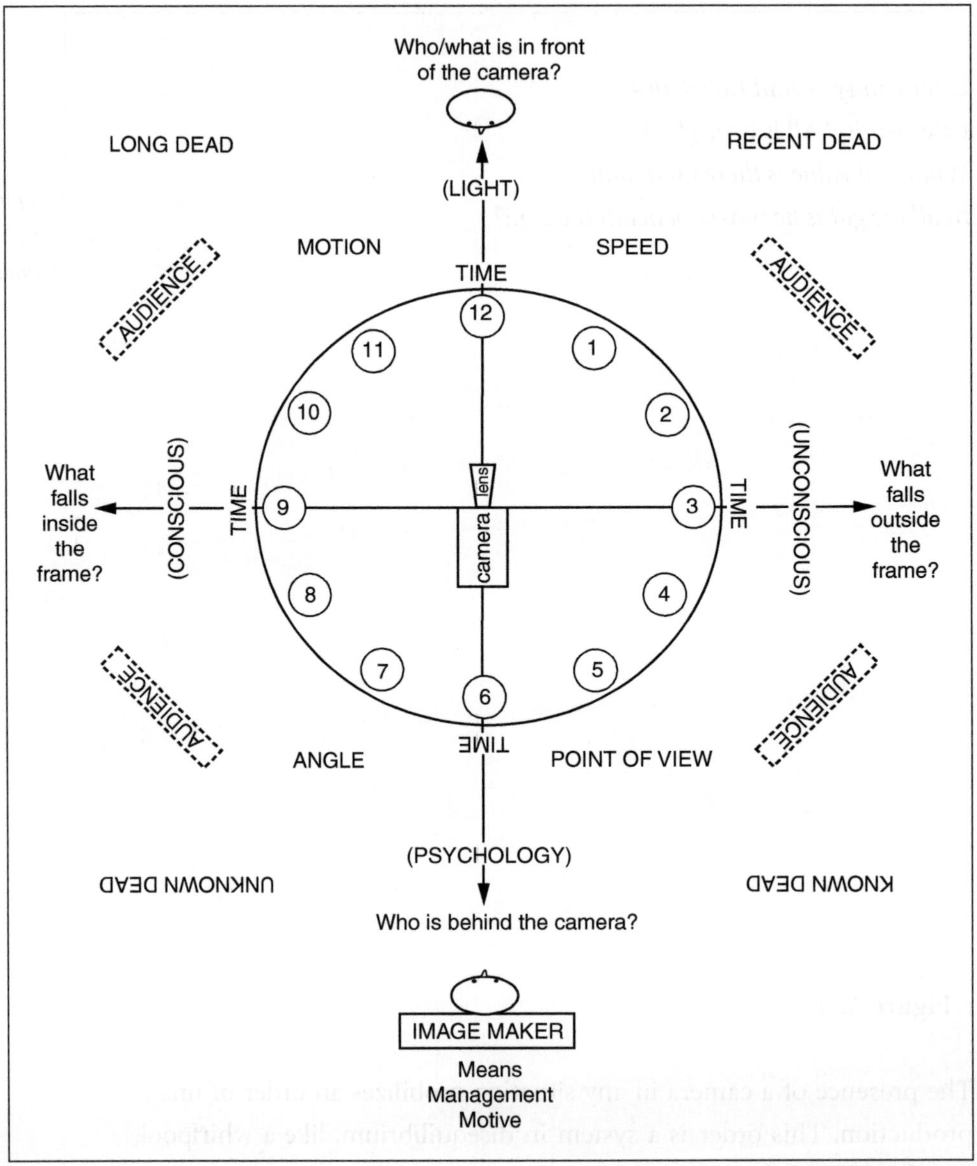

Figure 13.1 *Figure A. The Order of Image Production.* © Gregg Bordowitz, 2003.

time-concept is more appropriate here. Time is not a consistent measure. Any single event can seem to happen in seconds, minutes, hours, days, and lifetimes. The clockface suggested in the figure has no hands.

Figure A.[2] is a snapshot of a constantly moving phenomenon. A useful picture, it enumerates the forces in play among a dynamic set of relations. The camera rests at the intersection of two perpendicular lines. The vertical line describes a continuum situated between the Image Maker looking through the eye-piece of the camera, and the person, or thing, observed standing in front of the camera.

The Image Maker has three primary concerns:

1. Motive: Where is the camera pointing and why?
2. Management: Are the camera and all the technical apparatus functioning optimally?
3. Means: Are there sufficient resources both technical and monetary to complete the production?

Capturing the drama of events is the job of the Image Maker. This occupation is a matter of psychology. Informed by his or her own motives, the Maker shines light on the person or object in front of the lens. Whatever stands there possesses its own psychological features. Its motives can only be partially comprehended by the observer. Some interests, desires, and qualities may be apparent, but psychological dimensions will always remain elusive.

2. The method used to draw this figure was derived from Susan Buck-Morss, *The Dialectics of Seeing: Walter Benjamin and the Arcades Project* (Cambridge, Mass.: The MIT Press, 1987), pp. 64–65. Buck-Morss demonstrates how Benjamin thought in coordinates, and she diagrams the dialectical image as the null point of two axes.

The vertical axis is crossed by another trajectory. The ends of the horizontal line are designated by two questions:

1. What falls inside the frame?
2. What falls outside the frame?

The inside of the frame is the domain of conscious thought. The outside is so vast that it's incomprehensible; it is similar in depth to the unconscious. The camera never rests easily between the two poles. The boundary between the conscious and the unconscious is porous.

Pivoting on an intersection, the camera encompasses the remaining coordinates of the scheme:

1. Motion: Any camera maneuver is choreographed in relation to the state of the thing glimpsed through the lens, whether it moves or reposes. When capturing movement one faces questions concerning light. These concerns are the same for moving pictures and still photography. A photograph is a moving image; its velocity is so slow that the image seems to be standing still. However, everything is in motion constantly and so every cameraperson must ask: Where is the source of light? Are artificial lights required? Conscious decision making governs the placement of light in a scene.
2. Speed is apprehended by variables of exposure to light. Here the aperture of the lens opens into the unconscious. The velocity of the animate world eludes any glimmer of reason. A blurred image introduces what the eyes can't grasp to what the mind dimly suspects: impermanence.
3. Angle: Where is the camera in relation to the horizon—high or low, level or slanted? The angle of the camera is a psychological con-

cern decided by the conscious consideration of the camera operator according to his or her interests: he or she asks, How is the person or object to be regarded by the viewer? How do we feel about it? Is it large or small? Can it be confronted directly, or do we encounter it through the corner of the eye? With the angle of the camera we are told how others view the object, or how the director wishes us to view it.

4. Point of view (POV): Who or what is looking through the camera? Using POV the camera takes on the role of a character with a psyche independent from both the camera operator and the viewer. POV is a psychologically motivated decision that shifts the perspective of the image into the realm of the unconscious. The camera as character, the camera as "I," the camera in the first-person invites the viewer to inhabit the psychic space of a fictional being. This allows the viewer to rely on his own feelings to understand the motives of a character. Though the viewer may know all the circumstances of the story, the character itself remains unaware of its own motives and the circumstances in which they arise.

The order of image production acknowledges that the audience is present before, during, and after the production. The audience includes the people appearing in the movie and those who recognize them. Everyone who watches the movie is part of its audience, even the dead. Dead people are a significant portion of the audience, and they're all pictured in figure A: those who died long ago and the recently deceased; dead people you knew personally and others who you never met.

Loss has a positive form. Anyone who has lost someone dear, or suffered the rejection of unrequited love, or tried to quit smoking, is intimately familiar with a significant absence that palpably inhabits the space around him, every moment, waking or sleeping. The substance of something-once-present-now-gone is material. It is no mere imagining. Rather, it takes physical form embodied in our relationships to ourselves and to others. To understand the substance of loss, we must first understand the person who suffers loss. The constituent elements of this subject are the core needs of its being: sustenance, both physiological and psychological—these two terms themselves are inseparable. They are not distinct categorically. Second, the subject cannot exist by him- or herself. He or she exists only in relation to others. Each person seeks sustenance from an other. Each individual must get and give nourishment and recognition from others and to others. Last, there is the medium of exchange among people. The matter of exchange is not only composed of the material exchanged. The exchange itself lends value to the nutrient elements that people give to each other. The value of the material given by a mother to a child, or from friend to friend, is determined by the importance a provider and a recipient have for each other. Values of importance are not equivalent or reciprocal among people in relationships. Each individual assigns a value of importance to people and objects according to the amount of dependence he or she has on them.[3]

So we depend on others. This is not news. What makes the schema intriguing is the way it plays out within a particular set of circumstances. For me the basic rules of the game were modified to fit the circumstances of an epidemic that implicated me and everyone I know. AIDS has been the singular object of fascination that arrested all other concerns. Responding to the particular demands of the crisis, I have worked through the human dramas in general: love, sex, friendship, vocation, and death.

3. See Andre Green's explication of Charles Sanders Pierce's notion of "thirdness" in *Andre Green at the Squiggle Foundation*, ed. Jan Abram (London and New York: Karnac Books, 2002), pp. 39–68.

[*Fast Trip, Long Drop* (1993)]

Fast Trip, Long Drop (*FTLD*) is a fifty-three-minute experimental autobiography, a collage of material drawn from years of activist video documentation and film archives. It was made at a very low point, when video activists were forced to rethink our practices because our strategies were exhausted. Until then, we had limited ourselves to showing positive images of people with AIDS (PWAs) "surviving and thriving." These strategies were legitimate responses to the overwhelmingly prejudicial representations of PWAs generated by the commercial media in the early days of the epidemic. Conditions changed. As Jean Carlomusto observed in the tape, the documentary footage of demos and actions that were once energizing became a source of sadness: a record of once-healthy now-dead friends and fellow activists. By the early nineties, PWAs and others in the communities hardest hit by AIDS needed something else. I needed something else. I needed to openly confront the burn-out and despair that many activists felt.

It was a period of hopelessness. The Berlin International AIDS conference had recently convened. Doctors announced to the world that no cure was on the horizon. (This was before the new treatments became available. Not that protease inhibitors are the cure.) I believed very strongly in the legitimating power of television and media, so it was important to me that the complexity of the AIDS crisis be represented from the point of view of a PWA directly addressing other PWAs. *FTLD* showed a group of people talking among themselves about coming to terms with the probability of death. This went against the grain of the almost mandatory hopefulness I adopted for my earlier work: affirmative tapes made at GMHC for people with HIV, like "Work Your Body" and "PWA Power." When I made *FTLD* I was tired of pretending for the sake of others that I would survive. I became preoccupied with the burdens that sick people bear on behalf of those around them who are well. I wanted to get a handle on despair and put it out there as a political problem to be recognized and discussed. If we couldn't do this, then we couldn't advance. I wanted to maintain a commitment to producing an *honest* media made in the interests of people living with AIDS. This necessitated a self-analysis and critique that led me into areas repressed or foreclosed by the earliest formulations of the mandate for AIDS-activist media.

FTLD was shot entirely in video with the exception of some appropriated historical footage, which was originally shot on film. The completed work was transferred to 16mm so it could be distributed as a film. *FTLD* was broadcast on television, but it was also screened in film festivals and had theatrical runs in New York, San Francisco, and other cities.

I revealed many details about my life in *FTLD:* my drinking; the story of my father's desertion; sex, including unsafe sex; feelings of intimacy and loneliness. When I was writing the script (*Dense Moments*) I wanted to become the protagonist of my own story; but I'm not a confessional artist. I used my own life as material to connect with a larger audience of people. I believed that if those experiences happened to me, they happened to a lot of people. I didn't and still don't think the experiences I talked about were special or unique. Wasn't that the point of coming out? To become identified with a common struggle? A common story? So, I included those bits of personal history as a way to tell a story shared by many.

A very important element of *FTLD* was the use of Klezmer music on the soundtrack, brilliantly composed and beautifully played by the Klezmatics.[4] I knew *FTLD* would have a Klezmer soundtrack before I knew

4. Klezmatics, *Jews with Horns* (Piranha[GEMA]/Psycho Freylekhs Music, 1994), Compact Disk. Nos. 6,7,9,11 commissioned by Gregg Bordowitz for his film *Fast Trip, Long Drop* (U.S.A., 1993).

anything else about the tape. I wasn't consciously aware of this at the time, but the intuitive choice of Klezmer referred to the fact that Jewishness was my first experience of otherness in the world. Jewishness was the background against which I understood otherness in general: I saw that the figure of the PWA was constructed as "other" in the same ways that Jews, women, people of color, queers and outcasts had been. Prejudice is a corrupt kind of logic, a kind of sick machine that enforces "normalcy" and profits by it at the expense of diversity and difference. Normalcy is a fiction like "the general public."

The choice of Klezmer was significant within the context of Jewish cultural politics. Klezmer is the product of Yiddish culture: Yiddish is the language of the diaspora. It's secular. Although there have been religious texts written in Yiddish, it was also the daily language of European and American Jewish life. It has a rich history of music, theater, literature, philosophy, and political thought. It was not, like Hebrew, the language of a modern Jewish state. Jewish identity is threefold: cultural, national, and religious. I identify most easily with the first, which I associate with Yiddish, and reluctantly with the second and third. I am very critical of Israel's policies and I am not religiously observant. I refuse to accept the nationalist character of Jewish identity as the sole determining feature of my Judaism. Working with the Klezmer music was a way to refer to a culture of survival developed in the diaspora.

I performed in *FTLD*. I appeared as myself in documentary footage from protests and in scripted scenes. I also took on the guise of a double named Alter Allesman, Yiddish for "old everyman." Splitting myself into two characters enabled me to act out versions of myself that I was afraid to show. I obviously had a desire to reveal them, but I needed a fictional ruse, a distancing device to remove myself from the pain and anguish I felt at the time. Inventing a double was a way to provoke skepticism in the audience about the veracity of the claims coming out of the author's mouth. Doubt can be productive; it forces people to wrestle with truth.

My work and life *depended* on the interrogation of truth claims. The claim that "AIDS is a death sentence" was effectively refused by my generation of AIDS activists. Many people died, many continue to die, but the refusal to accept that "AIDS is a death sentence" led to the development of treatments prolonging my life and the lives of others. My peers and I were encouraged by our student readings of Michel Foucault to fight against the death sentence of AIDS. Foucault taught us to reject the authoritarian gaze of the medical profession. We elevated ourselves to the status of experts on the subject of AIDS. We learned from Foucault's method. When he analyzed penal institutions, he listened to prisoners, not their jailers. Interrogating mental institutions, he attended to the needs of patients rather than the psychiatrists. Following these examples, we struggled to give voice to people with AIDS. The idea that truth is a field of contestation gave us more than a tactical approach to our activism: it gave us hope.

FTLD was charged with a vitality that often bordered on hysteria. It drew its energy from panic and fear of death, certainly, but there was more than that. There was a clinging-to-life, a love-of-living, a wanting-more. An artist must do more than mobilize doubt and skepticism if the work of art is to yield its full potential for new articulations. To raise doubts productively one must situate the inquiry against a backdrop of wonder. I agree with the twentieth-century Jewish theologian, Abraham Heschel, that "Doubts may be resolved, radical amazement can never be erased. There is no answer in the world to man's radical wonder. Under the running sea of our theories and scientific explanations lies the aboriginal abyss of radical amazement."[5]

5. Abraham Heschel, *Man Is Not Alone* (New York: Noonday, 2000), p. 13.

The editing of *FTLD* is paced to feel breathless, exuberant. The ideas rush forward. It drew its momentum from an underlying desperation for answers to difficult questions: Why is this happening to me and the people around me? Where will this end? No definitive conclusion could be drawn, and yet the vitality of the inquiry implied hope for the future. *FTLD* was rushing toward something: its desperation was countered by a belief in something better.

FTLD was formulated to include despair and mourning within a political framework of analysis. To resist the conclusions drawn from the logical end of profound despair, a kind of nihilism, I marshaled a set of emotional strategies for coping with loss. In *FTLD* I tried to produce as many moments as possible where the viewer didn't know whether to laugh or cry. The emotional cues were inconclusive, hybrid. Emotional confusion opens up the possibility for a new landscape of affects, a terrain of unexplored sensations. Cliché and canned sentimentality may provide comfort in the short term, but ultimately it deadens our capacity to feel.

The Brechtian approach famously embraces shock as a mobilizing inducement to see the world anew. *FTLD* was crafted with Brecht in mind. Defamiliarization was its goal. For me, shock and astonishment are intimately linked. I'm concerned with what occurs immediately after the moment of a shocking rupture within the present actuality. The instance of surprise that interrupts the continuity of perception, so vital to the maintenance of consciousness, should not easily resolve itself into any one emotion—fear or anger, joy or calm. It should not come to rest around a particular object of contemplation. If a feeling of awe is produced, divorced from a particular emotion or object, it will linger in the mind of the viewer; the defamiliarization will continue after the film is over. Again, Heschel is instructive here: "What fills us with radical amazement is not the relations in which everything is embedded but the fact that even the minimum of perception is a maximum of enigma. The most incomprehensible fact is the fact that we comprehend at all."[6]

Two assumptions are key to understanding my work: First, we can make choices. To a large extent our actions are determined by numerous conditions—biological, psychological, and social. And yet I affirm that there is an arena of practical consciousness in which our choices are unfettered; and they matter. Second, I believe there is genuine novelty in the world. The question of novelty is fraught with contradiction because the production of novelty is an engine for consumer culture. Much of what is presented as new and improved is neither. In spite of capitalism's homogenizing effects, truly new things, conditions and relations do arise.

In *FTLD,* characters spoke directly to the camera as a means to play with the audience's various identifications. One speaking subject addressed the camera from a specific identity location—as a person with AIDS, for example—only to be replaced by another subject identifying from an entirely different location. In this way, the movie provokes members of the audience to contemplate how they speak about themselves, and how they feel about others' articulations. The conceptual motor for this exercise was Jacques Lacan's theory of the mirror stage. Lacan advanced the idea that the infant misrecognizes himself for the image in the mirror. Self-image and identity are necessary fictions. Acknowledging their fictional nature does not mitigate their significance, however. People are willing to die defending their allegiances.

Large sections of *FTLD* were structured like run-on sentences. The edits were not cuts, but conjunctions. An identity claim was advanced and then canceled by the following assertion. The claims were linked together in long chains. The formulation looked something like this: I am sick, but

6. Ibid., p. 14.

I am well, and I am gay, and proud, but angry, and confused; and I'm Jewish, but secular, and I have AIDS, which is not my fault, but I feel ashamed; I am alone, yet not entirely alone . . . Identities are most interesting when they're burdened to the point of collapse.

The underlying structure that served as the support for a seemingly haphazard construction was the result of years of television watching. When I watch TV, I don't watch one program. I surf the channels. Television is a cosmos in itself. The potential for recombination of its elements seems infinite.

When I was first formulating the ideas behind *FTLD,* I played games with the television. I flipped rapidly through the channels, writing down fragments of spoken words. The chance arrangement of phrases often yielded powerful poetic fragments. This game made me giddy.

Another game I used to play was "find the Nazi." The first thing I would do when I turned the television on was flip around until I found a historical representation—from a documentary, drama, or comedy—that depicted an image of a man in a Nazi uniform. It never failed. No matter what time of day, I could always find a Nazi on television. I didn't know what it meant, but the discovery was horrifying. I don't know if this game works anymore: I stopped playing it ten years ago.

FTLD is designed to approximate the experience of cycling through the channels of television in three complete revolutions during one hour of viewing. The body of the video is built around a spiral of three overlapping, equally proportioned circles. This is illustrated in figure B. The circles are clock faces, oriented differently in space. Each is segmented into fragments of several programs. Many of the common forms of television programming are parodied: news, talk show, documentary, drama, public service announcements. Each fragment was timed to last around three to four minutes, except for the public service announcements, which lasted

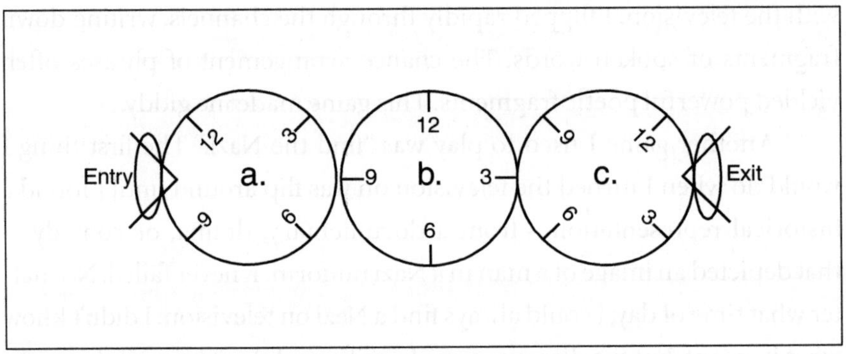

Figure 13.2 *Figure B. The Structure of* Fast Trip, Long Drop. © Gregg Bordowitz, 2003.

only a minute. To increase the velocity of the tape, I tried not to let any single shot exceed thirty seconds. In the end, I violated all the rules of the game, but the guidelines informed the basic timing and rhythm of the work. Once the spiral form was adopted and plotted, the problem of entry and exit had to be solved. I bracketed the tape with an introduction and a conclusion. The entry and exit are elliptical. They begin and end abruptly with the feeling that something's been omitted.

Walter Benjamin's writings influenced the making of *FTLD* enormously. I carried a photocopy of his "Theses on the Philosophy of History"[7] in my pocket. At the end of the "Theses," Benjamin observed that the Jew lives in an anticipatory present. Each moment, he wrote, is "the strait gate through which the Messiah might enter."[8] Benjamin was talking about a consciousness of time among a diasporic people who had suffered greatly through history. He said (this is my paraphrase, my understanding): "Look at the Jews. The Jews have a different sense of time. Throughout their struggles and wanderings, they hold out for the possibility of change, always in the present." This waiting creates a kind of character, a way of living, a way of thinking about possibility. Not that redemption will come in the hereafter. Redemption may come at any moment, here and now, in the historical present. Benjamin proposed this as one way of thinking about Marxist revolutionary struggle. The revolutionary is not content to wait for deliverance; he must work to bring about positive change. This is an argument for agency. The contradictions of capitalism will not inexorably lead to its collapse. The oppressed will not overcome their subjugation through some law of history guaranteed by transcendental forces, or

7. Walter Benjamin, "Theses on the Philosophy of History," *Illuminations,* ed. Hannah Arendt, trans. Harry Zohn (New York: Schocken Books, 1968), pp. 253–264.
8. Ibid., p. 264.

materialist principles. The patient and consistent activism of the oppressed is required for liberation to occur.

The notion of an anticipatory present spoke to the experience of people living with AIDS. We lived moment to moment waiting for the miraculous appearance of a cure. The character of our restless waiting called to my mind the image of Benjamin's long-suffering European Jew as the model revolutionary.

[*A Cloud in Trousers* (1995)]

And I feel
"I"
is too small for me.
Some other body is bursting out.[9]

One final image haunted the structure of *FTLD*. Deep in the back of my mind I must have retained the image of Tatlin's *Monument to the Third International* with its ever-narrowing spirals leading upward, reaching for the sky.

After *FTLD*, I shot my first work on 16mm film titled *A Cloud in Trousers*. The thirty-five-minute film is a staged reading of the great Soviet poet Vladimir Mayakovsky's famous poem, written in 1914–1915. It was an attempt to go beyond the autobiographical mode of *FTLD* by appropriating the allegorical potential of another artist's work. Mayakovsky's poem is lyrical and didactic, romantic and materialist. It swings pendulously between two equally passionate commitments: political revolution and

9. Vladimir Mayakovsky, "A Cloud in Trousers," *Twentieth Century Russian Poetry*, eds. John Glad and Daniel Weissbrot (Iowa City: University of Iowa Press, 1992), p. 13.

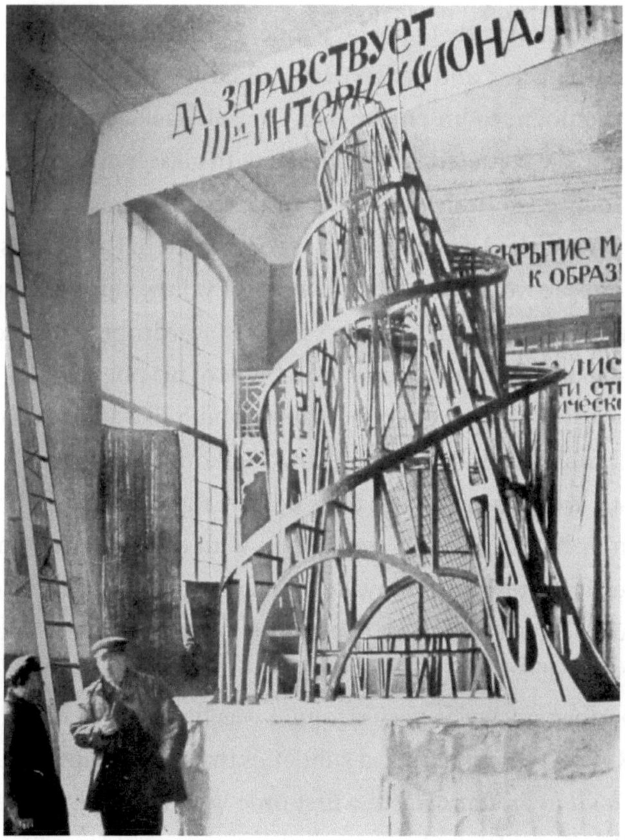

Figure 13.3 Vladimir Tatlin, model of the *Monument to the Third International,* at an exhibition in Moscow in 1920. Tatlin is in the foreground holding a pipe. Illustration from Ivan Puni's book *Tatlin* (Protiv Kubizma, 1931). © Private collection/Bridgeman Art Library.

romantic love. The dynamic tension in the poem emanates from a conflict. The poet wishes for social transformation with every fiber of his being. But the revolution is a demanding lover: it requires the withdrawal from all other romantic interests. It demands fidelity. The suspension of one's own amorous desires for the sake of a greater commitment is a theme that speaks most directly to my own inner conflicts.

I cast the actor and writer David Rakoff to play Mayakovsky declaiming the poem to an empty bar. The set was basically a black box. There were a few scattered tables littered with glasses and bottles. Most of the shots focused entirely on Rakoff and a chair set beside him. He wore a simple suit adorned with a wooden spoon stuck in the jacket's lapel as a boutonniere. He wore a top hat and a bright yellow shirt. The spoon and the hat were details of Mayakovsky's Futurist wardrobe taken from an account recorded in an introduction to a book of his poetry.[10]

Mayakovsky was over six feet tall and built like a boxer. He was macho and famously good-looking. David Rakoff does not have the same physical stature as the poet, nor does he have the manner of a boxer. He is an extremely handsome and gentle man with distinctly Jewish features. My choice of casting him as Mayakovsky had to do with my own desires—what I found commanding and beautiful. I wasn't trying to approximate some version of Mayakovsky: I wanted to make my own Mayakovsky. David's performance was very strong. I was happy with it. It's a difficult text and it required nuances and subtleties that David captured.

A Cloud in Trousers was the first time I worked with a cinematographer—Ellen Kuras. We had one day to shoot, so we met several times before that day to loosely storyboard the film. We looked at a lot of Rodchenko

10. Patricia Blake, ed., "Introduction: The Two Deaths of Vladimir Mayakovsky," *The Bedbug and Selected Poetry* (Cleveland and New York: Meridian Books, 1960), pp. 9–50.

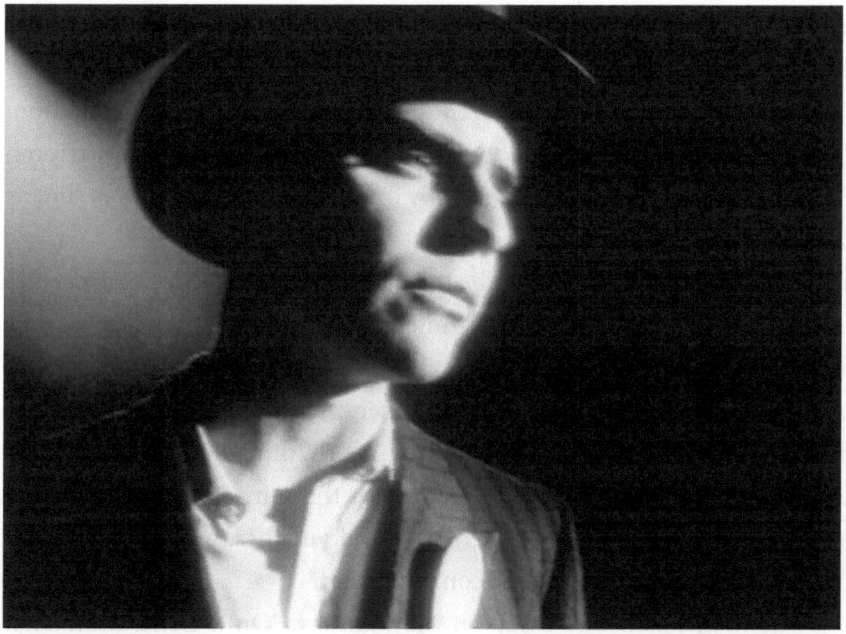

Figure 13.4 David Rakoff as Mayakovsky, in Gregg Bordowitz, *A Cloud in Trousers*, 1995.

photographs. When we got on the set, Ellen, who had far more experience shooting a film than anyone else, generously lent her expertise and enthusiasm to the enormous effort required. We had one day to complete the entire shooting schedule. I concentrated on David's performance and looked through the lens weighing different camera options Ellen offered me.

The film was shot in ways that enabled me to edit the material with continuity, although in the editing I chose to break with some rules of continuity, including jump cuts for the sake of rhythm. We did long takes starting on the darkness of the set's backdrop and ending on blackness. This allowed me to marry different takes and use black as punctuation. The camera was often but not always handheld. When using a tripod, Ellen usually moved the camera. Only one section of the film was shot as a series of portrait-like shots using a static camera.

The film was designed to be the meeting point of three distinct elements motivated by three separate intentions. David Rakoff's choices motivated the performance. The camera itself was established as a character struggling between interest and indifference. Finally, the third source of intention was embodied in the editing. Its rhythms did not necessarily match the rhythms of the performance or the camera work. Of course, the rules weren't strictly adhered to in the end, and there are junctures in the film where the three intentions come together.

Roman Jakobson's essay on Mayakovsky, "On a Generation That Squandered Its Poets,"[11] was very important to my understanding of Mayakovsky and the problems his generation of poets faced: the disillusionment and despair following the end of a political movement and its

11. Roman Jakobson, "On a Generation That Squandered Its Poets," *Language In Literature* (Cambridge, Mass. and London, England: Belknap Press of Harvard University Press, 1987), pp. 273–300.

subsequent calcification into a repressive bureaucracy. I projected my own concerns on to the poem, my feelings of loss and frustration about the AIDS movement. It was willful on my part. Specious, perhaps. This projection allowed me to explore how AIDS had distorted my sense of self. I felt reduced to my own creation: the persona of a diseased man. I felt that the first-person subject of my autobiographical work as a person with AIDS—my "I"—was "too small for me." "Some other body was bursting out."

The aesthetic problems of political art issue out of an oscillation between two poles. On the one hand there are formal preoccupations and commitments drawn and inspired by the exigencies of politics. On the other hand there are subjective desires issuing from an irrational psychic core, the sources of which are the constitutional conflicts of the individual. Jakobson wrote:

> Formalist literary theory placed the lyric monologue in quotes and disguised the "ego" of the lyric poet under a pseudonym. But what unbounded horror results when suddenly you see through the pseudonym, and the phantoms of art invade reality. . . .[12]

[*The Suicide* (1996)]

The tensions arising between the demands of AIDS activism and my increasing desire to explore aspects of my life outside the framework of AIDS resulted in the appropriation of another work from the Soviet avant-garde: Nicolai Erdman's play *The Suicide.* The plight of Semyon, the main character, spoke to me. Semyon tries to unyoke himself from the

12. Ibid., p. 293.

enforced optimism of a bureaucratic order that prohibits any discussion of disappointment and despair following the revolution:

> Dear God! Have we done anything against the revolution? From the very first day have we ever done anything against it? We visit each other and we tell each other that life is hard, because life is easier when you can say that it is hard.[13]

I often refer to my adaptation of *The Suicide* as my Waterloo. A hugely ambitious project, it was a campaign that failed owing to a lack of resources and a gross underestimation on my part of the effort's requirements. The source text for the movie was brilliant. It was so incisive in its critique that Stalin banned *The Suicide* while it was in rehearsal at Meyerhold's theater in 1932. A corrosive comedy about the shortcomings of the Bolshevik revolution, the story follows the misadventures of the unemployed protagonist, Semyon Semyonovich Podsekalnikov, who threatens to kill himself because he has no livelihood. When word gets out through gossipy neighbors that he's threatened suicide, representatives of various interests approach him and ask him to kill himself on their behalf. An intellectual inspires him to kill himself in the name of the Russian intelligentsia. A romantic seduces him to kill himself for love. A butcher begs him to kill himself over the high price of meat! No one tries to save him.

My ninety-minute adaptation of the comedy addressed the concerns of political art after the fall of Soviet Communism. I wanted to make a post–Cold War movie. It was a redemptive effort: saving the work of an artist who suffered under Stalin's thumb. At the same time, I wanted to redeem the losses of those who suffered from anti-Communist persecution

13. Nikolai Erdman, *The Suicide*, trans. Peter Tegel (London: Pluto Plays, 1981), p. 52.

in the United States, particularly the victims of McCarthyism. With all that in mind, I decided to produce a movie adaptation of *The Suicide* as if it were a live broadcast production on American television of the fifties. I became obsessed with the phenomenon of live drama on broadcast television. I spent hours at the Museum of Broadcasting in New York City, watching kinescopes of live productions for television: *Requiem for a Heavyweight, Marty, The Comedian, The Last Tycoon* and *The Days of Wine and Roses,* among many others.

Live drama for television represented a short-lived utopian moment in the history of the medium, when television was still experimental. Produced out of New York City, drawing on the talents of the city's stages, employing actors trained in "the method" and writers who faced the blacklist in Hollywood, live televised theater was gritty, realist, populist, and progressive. Formally, it was unique—a hybrid of film, theater, and television. The broadcasts had the ambition and seriousness of cinema, plus the excitement of live performance, all scaled down to fit on a tiny screen set into a piece of living room furniture.

With my production of *The Suicide,* I set out to collapse the false antinomies of the Cold War—America the "land of the free" versus Russia the "evil empire"—into one bizarre and freakish object. I succeeded at that. Using a small inheritance from my grandparents, I took a cast and crew down to the Wexner Center for the Arts, in Columbus, Ohio. The Wexner Center granted me a residency, allowing me to shoot and edit the production at their facilities. We built three nineteen-twenties period sets in different areas of the Wexner, and costumed all the actors in period clothing.

I worked with cinematographer Ben Speth to approximate the production methods of a fifties television studio. We used two separate video cameras on tracks. The actors' movements were choreographed with the cameras' movements. The actors and the camera operators each had established marks to hit precisely at different moments during the dialogue. The scenes ran long, some twenty minutes in length or more. I established the rule that once I yelled "Action!" the actors couldn't stop regardless of what happened. I told them that they should proceed as though the taping were a live broadcast. If they flubbed a line, they had to recover as if they were on stage in front of a live audience. (I purposely cast actors with theater experience.) Although I did have a chance to rehearse with the actors in New York before arriving in Columbus, we didn't have money to build sets in New York, so we had to wait to block the scenes in the Wexner studio before we shot them.

There was an extra-added pressure. I had only ten days to shoot the entire thing. We completed production on schedule. Everyone left Columbus. I stayed behind to edit the ninety-minute rough cut in one week. To this day the reasons behind this maniacal undertaking defy explanation.

The Suicide was shot and edited using conventional rules of narrative continuity. The work was an experiment in medium hybridization and genre mixing. It remains an interesting work (for me), but it's compromised. The sound quality is uneven and so is the cinematography. There are good performances and embarrassing performances. Ultimately, it actually looks like a live telecast. Even during the heyday of broadcast drama, the productions could be clumsy and unpolished. However, it was the masterpieces of the genre that inspired me. John Frankenheimer's *The Comedian* was the model. Unfortunately, my work fell far short of the excellence his model exemplified.

Still, *The Suicide* was a good vehicle to explore issues surrounding the burdens placed on "victims" by society. PWAs were held responsible for burdens on the health care system. We were blamed for the collapse of the

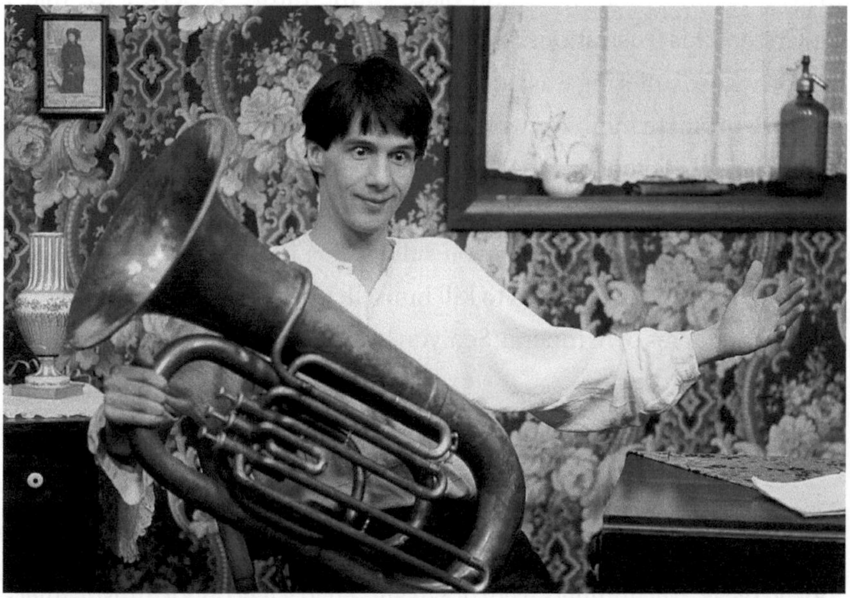

Figure 13.5 Lothaire Bluteau as Semyon, in Gregg Bordowitz, *The Suicide,* 1996.

nation's moral order. We placed burdens on the legal system. We ruined sex. We were a blank wall upon which many ills could be projected according to the cynical interests of various parties. Conversely, PWAs were also made the subjects of fantasies from within the AIDS movement. We were turned into angels and heroes.

Semyon is an unemployed man in a society promising full employment. He lived through the revolution and expected to benefit from it. Instead he finds that he has no place in the future society. I felt that I understood his frustrations. I saw Semyon as a person living with AIDS. A person whose suffering was turned into a political football. My adaptation is a post-protease inhibitor work. My interest in the play and mining it for its allegorical content had to do with the realization that I might live much longer than I had expected.

Out of desperation, Semyon offered his life as a martyr to many causes. In the end, he refused to kill himself. He wanted to live. In his final monologue at his own funeral, Semyon begs everyone to allow him to live.

[*Habit* (2001)]

At the moment, I am fairly healthy. There was a period, in 1993, when things looked bleak. My numbers were down and I had a few opportunistic infections. Fortunately, the infections could be treated and I was able to maintain my health until the protease inhibitors came around in 1995. I went on a cocktail and my health improved. I'm doing well on the new drugs, and now I have to face the fact that I may live for a long time. But underneath all this optimism is the lingering fear that I'm fooling myself. That the drugs will stop working and I'll become resistant to all available treatments. A likely outcome. So my health, my life, my plans, continue to be provisional.

It's difficult for me to talk about longevity. I've lost many friends and I feel that I owe it to them not to complain about living. After all, living longer, surviving, does not fall into the category of oppression. I'm lucky, right? However, I tested positive when I was twenty-three. I didn't think I was going to be living in two years. Forget living to see thirty. I spent my entire twenties thinking I was going to die. I didn't prepare for a long life. I gave no thought to money or a career. I didn't think about what I wanted to do with my life, or rather I did: I decided that I would do only what was meaningful to me in the short time that I thought I had. Now I find myself facing the more abstract questions of existence like, what do I want to do for the rest of my life? I feel like a child sometimes.

Habit is a sequel to *FTLD.* It's a fifty-two-minute autobiographical documentary that follows the current events of the AIDS epidemic along several trajectories. The organizing structure is built around my daily routine. As I move through the day, attending to mundane errands, eating, taking pills, having conversations with friends (some who have diseases like AIDS and breast cancer, and others who are healthy), memories of a recent trip to South Africa recur and interrupt the routine.

In July, 2000, I went to Durban, South Africa to attend the International Conference on AIDS. I met people with AIDS fighting to get access to the same life-saving drugs that I depend on to survive. The documentary *Habit* records the efforts of South Africa's leading AIDS activist group, the Treatment Action Campaign (TAC), struggling to gain access to these drugs. Running parallel to this documentation, there is a rigorous working through of ideas concerning privilege, ethics, responsibility, futility, solidarity, hope, and struggle. The most challenging and the most urgent aspect of this new work is the sense of responsibility that arose from making the tape: to do whatever I can to help those who do not have access to the same drugs that keep me and my friends alive.

Unfortunately, there is little I can do to help the millions of people without proper care and treatment. I do what I can and I go about the business of my own life. Habit is the substance of daily life. Our lives are defined by daily activities that are often rendered invisible or unremarkable through repetition. In the video, I embrace the notion of habit. I do not reject it as deadening or stultifying. Habit is understood as the backdrop against which epiphany arises. Genuine novelties—new things, new relations—are identified by the remarkable qualities that make them profoundly different from the features of the quotidian. The continual performance of habits establishes the continuity necessary to sustain our sense of coherence about the world we inhabit. The repetitive nature of daily existence allows for the incorporation of new features into our lives through habit. Habit is the medium of experience. The awe that novelty evokes can be faced only when it is tamed and captured by habit. The oscillation between habit and wonder is the space of potential. We need both poles. Without wonder we are enslaved to conformity. Without habit we have no continuity. This conclusion is disappointing. The "revolutionary" will refuse submission to conformity and continuity. The "conformist" will feel undermined by the admission that chance always destroys the best-laid plans. I have sympathy for both of you. I am both a revolutionary and a conformist. This conundrum cannot be resolved in favor of one or the other. We each resolve it by modifying the proportion of one impulse to the other.

The tape is organized into three sections, or movements, like a piece of chamber music. The three sections explore the themes of habit, foreignness, and intimacy. The first ten minutes of the tape present a meditation on waking up and the habits that constitute the morning: hygiene, breakfast, pill-taking, and yoga. It contrasts my morning with my girlfriend's. Although I talk about my bisexuality in *FTLD,* people are often

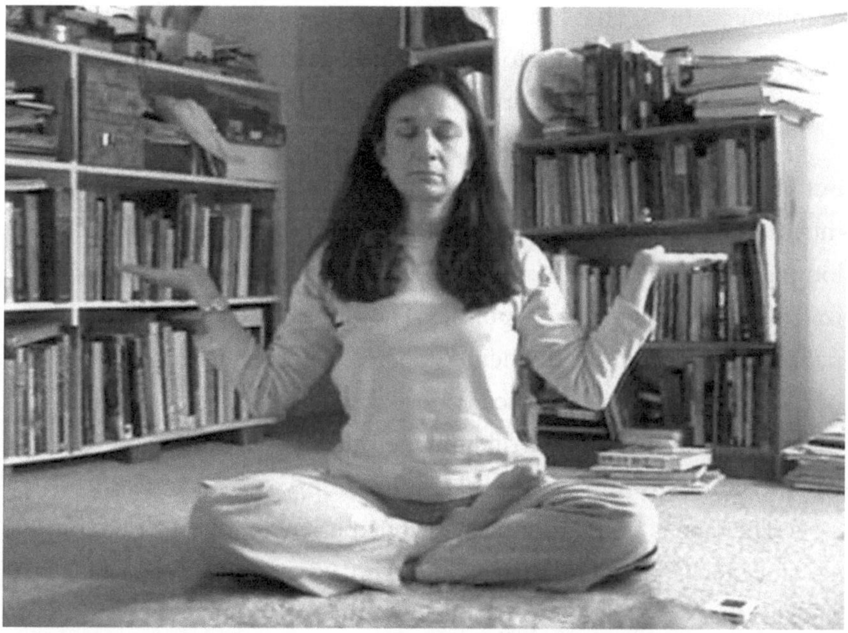

Figure 13.6 Claire Pentecost. From Gregg Bordowitz, *Habit,* 2001.

surprised to see that I am in a domestic, erotic, and amorous relationship with a woman. Claire Pentecost and I have been together for nine years. Among the habits I don't discuss in the tape is our sex life. I don't explore this for a couple of reasons. First, out of respect for Claire's privacy. Not everyone has the perverse need to expose the intimate details of their life in video. Second, because I have addressed matters of sex and sexuality rigorously in many previous works and I wanted here to focus on other mundane matters. That I consider sex a routine matter is a feature of age. Sex is no longer mysterious to me. Sex is not a panacea. It can be great. It's often good, sometimes perfunctory; occasionally, it makes me sad.

Perhaps I should have dealt with issues of HIV prevention in *Habit,* but I found the issues concerning treatment access so overwhelming and intricate that I needed to limit my focus. And there are other reasons. I long ago stopped trying to reconcile my life experiences with the authorized narratives of movement politics. The names used to describe our sexualities are impoverished when compared with the actual messiness of our sexual lives. Object choice is beyond volition. The preference for a lover becomes an existential dilemma only in the sense that we can choose whether or not to embrace the selections our psyches make for us.

The tape is built around my own experiences. I haven't had unsafe sex since 1993. I'm not boasting and I'm not complaining. I just can't bear the idea that I could be responsible for another person's infection. Sometimes, I wish I could; but I can't. Frankly, I am stumped when it comes to saying anything new about sex and self-care—I have many thoughts, but nothing solid has formed yet: I suspect that issues around sex and volition as they pertain to prevention will be the subject of my next work.

In contrast to the first part of the tape's examination of habit, the second section is organized around the idea of foreignness. It consists of material shot entirely in South Africa, depicting the work of HIV-positive activists. This section juxtaposes three different situations regarding treatment. Edwin Cameron, a white High Court Justice testifies to the life-saving role treatment plays in his life. Promise Mthembu, a TAC activist and mother, talks about the difficulty she has obtaining medical treatment. Finally, Zackie Achmat, the chairperson of the TAC, explains why he refuses to take HIV medicines until they are available to all the citizens of South Africa who need them. All three testimonies are very painful and moving.

The first two sections together establish a dichotomy between "here" and "there." A number of questions inform this inquiry: how can people who exist across great divides of geography and resources have meaningful relationships? How can we join our efforts to address structural inequities implicit to global capitalism? Here is a simple truth we all live with: our good fortune and luxurious lifestyles in the United States are provided for us at the expense of those who live and work in poverty "elsewhere." I wanted to think in a rigorous way about this fundamental contradiction without necessarily lapsing into a facile discussion organized around blame. I live a very comfortable life. I have access to life-saving drugs available to only a fraction of the world's HIV-positive population. The benefits I enjoy are the result of a vast global economy; they are impersonal. In other words, there is nothing special about me that grants me access to resources. I am simply very fortunate to have found myself in these circumstances. Where lies my responsibility? What can I do from this vantage to help others? What do others want of me? What do they expect from me? I tried to ask these questions without resorting to a guilt trip, which is very counterproductive. Guilt makes people shut down. I wanted to openly discuss privilege. To admit that I have it and to wonder aloud about what I should do with it.

Another aspect of the video is that I refused to represent the South Africans as "victims." All of my AIDS work has rejected the role of victim for PWAs. I did not want the story I'm telling to fall into a simplistic narrative that produces an emotional experience solely for the enjoyment of viewers removed from the irresolvable difficulties of the situation. The Africans in my tape are fighting for their lives. They have dignity and poise. They provide us with a cogent analysis of global capitalism and the workings of the pharmaceutical industry. I didn't have to go to Africa to see crushing poverty, or to talk to people without access to health care and drugs. I can go to neighborhoods where I live in Chicago to find that. In South Africa, I encountered an AIDS movement with a compelling global analysis and exciting ideas about how to fight AIDS on a global scale. One of the things I'm thinking about lately is how the current focus of attention on Africa, and the problem of poverty in the third world, has eclipsed the problems of poverty at home.

When I was in South Africa I tried to assimilate the demonstrations I witnessed into my own past experiences with protests. On a TAC-organized march through the streets of Durban I felt nostalgia for the eighties activism of ACT UP. In Durban there were 5,000 people wearing t-shirts with the words "HIV positive" boldly printed on their chests. I felt the urge to say, "Wow, this is 1989. This is just like 1989 was for us." Of course, that is enormously arrogant and not correct. I had to think that through and I realized that the African situation is singular. It has its own integrity, its own logic. Undeniably, there is a shared history of activism around the world, and at the same time there are unassimilable differences between situations of crisis. In South Africa the well-informed core leadership of TAC has read Douglas Crimp's work. It has followed ACT UP's history. It has borrowed articulations and signage from all over the globe. Similarities were the first points of entry for me, but they do not yield the deepest understanding. I don't know what it is like to live in a place where one out of three people have HIV, as it is in some places in Africa. I've been to a lot of funerals, too many, and yet I don't know what it is like to attend funerals daily. And finally, I don't know what it is like to face this disease without some measure of security.

It's facile to reconcile foreign situations with your own. On a philosophical level, one must admit that everything is made of the same substance. That's a very simple verity and everyone can agree with that. But what is different about things? Each thing is the same as another in some respect and profoundly different in other ways. One must work hard *not* to lose the differences, the novel aspects that can alter and expand one's consciousness.

The juxtapositions of habit and foreignness, "here" and "there," funnel into the third section of the tape. (See Figure C.) The last thirty minutes of *Habit* is organized around the concept of intimacy. The video has a formula, a proposition: the reconciliation of habit and foreignness is intimacy. This reconciliation is not fully achieved in life and so the tape ends on an uneasy feeling of irresolution. Of what does intimacy consist?

The substance of intimacy is love. We can overcome great divisions through chosen affiliations. A cold materialism theorizes that alliances are formed solely around interests. There's truth in that. Interests often determine alliances, but common interests are not enough to explain why we choose to link our struggles to others', or why we adopt others' struggles as our own.

The long section on intimacy in *Habit* is broken up by three interventions. The first is an interview with Claire Pentecost in her studio. It's a meditation on interiority: the interior life is affirmed as a necessary and inescapable condition. The second is a meditation on the continuity between the mind and the body. Yvonne Rainer and I compare notes about aging and illness. Yvonne teaches me that "My body is the only reality." The third intervention concerns spirituality. For this consideration, I interviewed my friends Richard Elovich and Daniel Wolfe, a gay couple who together enjoy spiritual practices such as meditation and prayer.

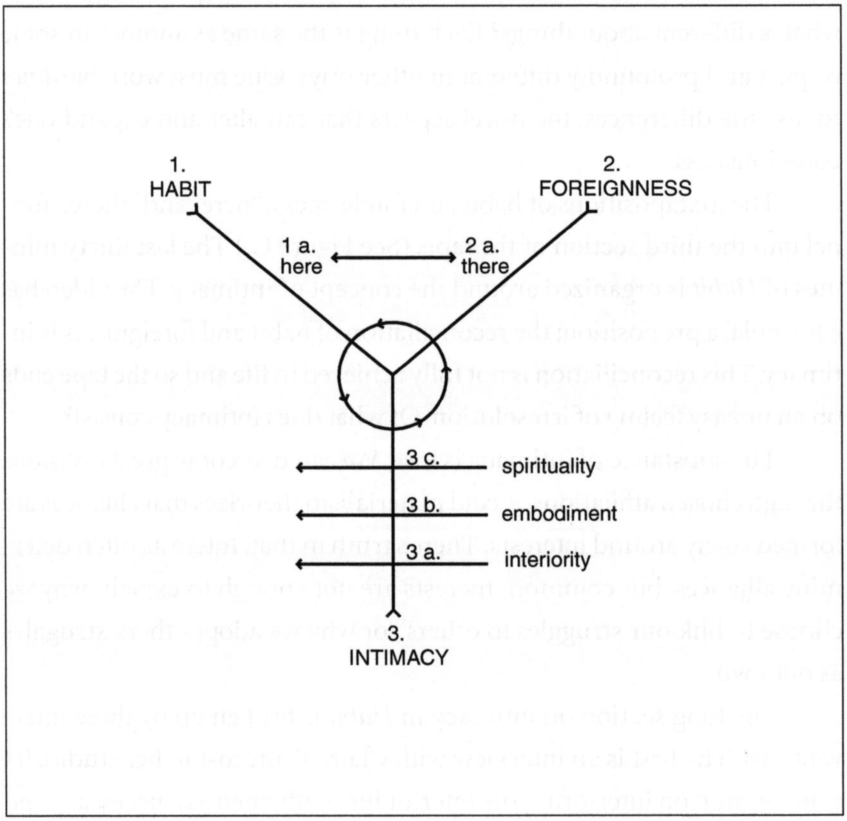

Figure 13.7 Gregg Bordowitz, *Figure C. The Structure of* Habit. © Gregg Bordowitz, 2003.

Daniel concludes that spiritual experiences are fragile; language threatens them with extinction.

Interiority, the body, and spirituality are three overlapping categories necessary to the investigation of subjectivity. What consitutes the subject? This is an enduring question informing my work. The inner life is a concept that has undergone much examination. The Romantic notion that we have vast inner worlds not readily available to others is a fundamental premise of modernism, regardless of whether it was embraced in part or rejected entirely by various artists.

The notion of the body, not the body itself, but the way we talk about it, structures much of our understanding of the relation between the self and others. HIV has placed the concern for the body and its representations at the center of my project.

Spirituality is a class of ideas, all bound together by the contention that there is something larger than the self governing the order of existence. Some people place their faith in a god. Some look to their relations with others to define their spirituality. One can reject all matters of religious belief and practice, yet still experience the yearning to be part of something large and meaningful that eludes description. Rather than contemplate a specific version of spirituality, I focused on the need for the category itself in the concluding section of *Habit.*

Intimacy is the sovereign principle governing human relations. Even hate is a kind of intimacy. I'm not trying to advance an Edenic ideal. Or perhaps, I am. There is a communitarian ideal underlying the videotape's inquiry into intimacy. I am preoccupied with ethical problems: How can we share resources? How can we meaningfully relate to each other, overcoming huge distances without erasing our differences?

The method of inquiry in *Habit* is significant. The ethical questions above are pursued through direct dialogue between myself and others.

The meditations on interiority, the body, and spirituality are all conducted as recorded conversations with my intimates.

Between the three interventions, I juggled interview material and recorded speeches showing people with AIDS addressing concerns of longevity, solidarity, hope, loss, and despair. All these elements are urgent concerns for each individual, with or without AIDS. They cause conflict and pain. My formula—habit plus foreignness equals intimacy—was a frustrated attempt to bring into harmony the discordant features of psychic life complicated by AIDS. The formula did not yield the reconciliation of "here" and "there" that I desired. I couldn't expect it to. Intimacy is an unresolvable dichotomy. One can not be an "I" without an Other, yet one can't fully become identical with an Other. Intimacy is a paradox. Being for the Other is an ethical ideal, absolutely necessary, fundamentally inescapable, and ultimately impossible.[14]

The problems of the AIDS pandemic are so complex that an end to the crisis is not immediately at hand. The problems are not resolvable in life, so they shouldn't be resolvable in a work of art. With *Habit,* as with all my films and videos, I aspired to make a political work of art: one that embodies in its form the ethical demands faced in our encounters with others as they arise out of current conditions of existence. To do this, I adhered to the following set of principles:

Political art produces irresolution.

Political art must adopt the imperatives of an activist movement as its starting point, not its end.

14. These ideas are inspired by, but not directly quoted from Levinas. See Emmanuel Levinas, *Ethics and Infinity: Conversations with Philippe Nemo,* trans. Richard A. Cohen (Pittsburgh: Duquesne University Press, 1982). Levinas insists on the irreducibility of the Other's alterity: "The pathos of the erotic relationship is the fact of being two, and that the other is absolutely other." Ibid., p. 66.

Political art is not supplemental to any cause. It is its own cause.

Political art does not earn its guarantee of relevance or truth from protests and activist efforts. Art must provide its own guarantees through form. The politics of art are not to be found anywhere but in the artwork itself.

Politics occur when the work of art is encountered in the here and now. Understand that the "here and now" is not entirely composed of the present moment. Rather, when a work of art is encountered, it draws force and substance from the dimension of the unconscious, which, as Freud instructed, is timeless. Works of art in general, and documentaries in particular, do not reconstruct events. They construct versions of past events informed by the present conditions of viewing and conjectures about future possibilities. All versions of events exist in potential for the observer engaging art. The encounter with art in the present involves intrapsychic operations, and so interpretation of the object is performed retrospectively after viewing. The time-concept for art is a non linear shuttling backward and forward. The job of the artist is to provide a biased ground for the construction of history, which is always alive and subject to change.

Political art must address questions of form. I advocate the crossbreeding of documentary procedures with poetry and the concerns of structure usually reserved for musical composition.

Politics is a matter of habit for me. Through mundane experiences I encounter an incomprehensible perplexity. The astonishment felt when facing novelty is both pleasurable and painful. Exceeding the limits of my worldview enriches my life. It reminds me that I've not yet reached my end. I'm still alive! At the same time it unsettles the semblance of continuity which I need for my consciousness to remain operational. There is a too-much-ness about the world around me. The senses have to filter out an enormous amount of sensation so that the body can focus on specific phenomena. At the same time, there is too much going on inside the body. We are all dimly aware of our physiological operations minute-to-minute.[15] Making *Habit* I became acutely aware of the pressure of external experience bearing down on my body and the pressure of internal experience bursting out of my body. If there is a provisional resolution at the end of *Habit,* I came to understand the notion of the subject, or individual, as a threshold, a limit-point, a boundary where contact and exchange between the inside and outside of experience meet.

I recall another time when that epiphany first enthralled me: the first time I took psychedelic mushrooms. My companion turned to me after what seemed to be a very long period of silence. With his eyes sparkling, he grinned as he said, "It's big out there." Though I was altered, my mind was unprepared to accept that truth. I wondered why he was smiling. I felt helpless.

The common word "helplessness" (*Hilflosigkeit* in German) is a significant reference-point in Freudian theory. It denotes

> the state of human suckling which, being entirely dependent on other people for the satisfaction of its needs (hunger, thirst), proves incapable of carrying out the specific action necessary to put an end to internal tension. For the adult, the state of helplessness is the prototype of the traumatic situation which is responsible for the generation of anxiety.[16]

15. See Brian Massumi, *Parables for the Virtual: Movement, Affect, Sensation* (Durham and London: Duke University Press, 2002). Massumi borrows many examples from science throughout his book to discuss the way the body must filter stimuli to produce a sense of coherence about the world. He also makes compelling arguments for the applicability of these ideas in the humanities.

16. J. Laplanche and J.-B. Pontalis, *The Language of Psychoanalysis,* trans. Donald Nicholson-Smith (New York and London: W. W. Norton, 1973), p. 189.

My dear friend Ray died twelve years ago. That's over twice the number of years we were friends. Still we remain close. His death preserved our friendship in a state of suspension. I feel like I continued to be Ray's friend without him, as if the friendship no longer required his presence. Or rather, his absence is a kind of presence.

When Ray was rendered blind and incapacitated by illness, I read sections of a book to him almost on a daily basis. The book was about a writer living among freedom fighters. They were gathered together in the desert awaiting the day when they would recapture their homeland. Maybe the book wasn't really about that at all. The story of a revolutionary struggle was the author's preoccupation. Yet, his underlying desires extracted their energy from another source. The writer longed for the maternal love denied to him in his infancy. His mother abandoned him for adoption. In his book, there is a recurring minor character, an older woman. The writer stayed once or twice as a guest in her home. She brings the author coffee one morning as he awakens in an unfamiliar bed, her son's bed. The woman is the mother of a soldier. Her son is away fighting in the desert. The author, Jean Genet, receives the coffee and in doing so becomes a substitute for the absent son. He and the mother act out their roles each fulfilling an obligation to another. Who knows what the book is actually about? For me this particular book will always be about my friend, the tragedy of his blindness and the opportunity I had to be present for him, sitting by his bedside reading aloud. The book's title is *Prisoner of Love.*[17]

I often looked at my friend with a mixture of awe and resentment. Sometimes, I hated the man lying in bed disabled by his disease. Or, was it the disease that I hated? I knew I loved Ray. I was confused and I remain confused. My own illness is no less mysterious to me than another's. I do

17. Jean Genet, *Prisoner of Love,* trans. Barbara Bray (London: Picador, 1989).

not identify with the "I" in the following sentence: I am ill. Who is it that has a disease? He is a stranger to me. His virus belongs to him.

[*Drive* (2002)]

> Vaughn died yesterday in his last car-crash. During our friendship he had rehearsed his death in many crashes, but this was his only true accident. Driven on a collision course towards the limousine of the film actress, his car jumped the rails of the London Airport flyover and plunged through the roof of a bus filled with airline passengers. The crushed bodies of the package tourists, like a haemorrhage of the sun, still lay across the vinyl seats when I pushed my way through the police engineers an hour later. Holding the arm of her chauffeur, the film actress Elizabeth Taylor, with whom Vaughn had dreamed of dying for so many months, stood alone under the revolving ambulance lights. As I knelt over Vaughan's body she placed a gloved hand to her throat.[18]

Rereading the first paragraph of Ballard's novel *Crash* brings my mind back to the early eighties, when I carried a dog-eared copy with me everywhere. The book was recommended reading in a college class on contemporary art taught by Sanford Kwinter. *Crash* spoke to me and my friends with its corrosive, Pop-inspired take on America-as-Hollywood-invention; a culture obsessed with sex, death, fame, and cars. For Ballard, the American body was an automobile and sex was a car crash. He saw the potential for

18. J. G. Ballard, *Crash* (New York: Vintage Books, Random House, 1985), p. 7.

technology as an extension of the human body. Machines embodied all the irrationality of the psyche.

Ballard grasps the affects of violence in a media-saturated culture. The spectacle of the accident is a medium for a volatile chemical reaction spewing off chunks of matter: metal, vinyl, skin, guts, and blood; organic and inorganic remnants alloyed into new compounds. Physics can't satisfactorily explain this event. Can a car wreck correctly be referred to as an accident? What role did the volition of the drivers play? Innocent victims never saw it coming. The damage is so extensive that no single witness can comprehend the cataclysm in its totality. The material is rich with allegorical potential. Even Elizabeth Taylor makes an appearance. The book was written in 1973, but Ballard couldn't possibly have known then that the movie star would later bear witness, as a charity organizer and fundraiser, to a catastrophe far greater than a car colliding with a bus.

The car is a vexing convenience. I didn't learn how to drive until I was thirty-six. For me, the car and the act of driving have always been freighted with painful associations. In 1976, my estranged biological father was killed in a freak accident, hit by a truck while walking on a country road. In 1980, I walked away shaken but unscathed from a collision. My stepfather was making a left turn off a highway. A speeding car coming from the opposite direction ploughed into our vehicle on my side just slightly behind me. The blow was absorbed by the frame between the front and back seats. I can still recall with great clarity the look of horror on the face of the other driver seconds before impact. That image is conjoined with the image of her bloodied and dazed face behind the fractured remaining shards of her windshield. In 1991, my paternal grandparents were killed when a truck collided with their car as they turned onto a highway exiting the parking lot of a pharmacy. These experiences accounted for the recurrent use of images depicting car crashes, crash tests and daring stunts by daredevils in *FTLD.* In *Habit,* the final title sequence began with an extended real-time shot, videotaped from the inside of a truck driving at night through the streets of Durban until it finally pulled into a parking garage. The shot ended when the truck came to rest in front of a sign: Dead Slow, Booms Ahead.

The image of the car returned in a gallery installation that was an element of my first one-person exhibition "Drive," at the Museum of Contemporary Art in Chicago, in 2002. The installation displayed a race-car covered with decals of the logos of every pharmaceutical company currently producing treatments for HIV disease. The car was an antique soap-box-derby car, built in the forties or earlier, approximately six feet in length and three feet in width, roughly the size of a coffin. The small opening in its body where the driver would sit was large enough to fit a ten-year-old. The car was pill-shaped, long, sleek and elliptical. For me, it was the essence of my modernity; the encapsulation of various traumas haunting me: road accidents, deaths, and pills.

I designed a pedestal for the car to capture the illusion of forward movement and to emphasize the feeling of velocity. It was a trapezoid, built slightly smaller than the length of the car and just wide enough to support the wheels. The top surface of the pedestal was painted a shade of gray blacktop. The sides were white, with a red racing stripe. The same vinyl stripe was applied all around the walls of the gallery and around the entryway of the room into the exhibition hall of the museum.

The gallery was roughly square, approximately twenty-four feet by twenty-four feet. A huge vinyl banner, twenty-two feet in length, was hung above the far wall. It declared in red letters on a yellow background: THE AIDS CRISIS IS STILL BEGINNING. On each side wall, an aluminum-framed clock was hung at the centerpoint of the walls. The two clocks faced each other. One was set to Chicago time, the other to Capetown time. The car and its pedestal were placed in the center of the room on a diagonal between the two clocks. A small cube in the corner of the room supported a stack of posters printed for the exhibition, available free to visitors.

The poster was printed on two sides of slick paper. The front had an illustration of the car and the logo designed for the exhibition. The design borrowed all the design conventions found in racing magazines. It listed the times and places of various events associated with the exhibition. I thought of the entire museum show as a campaign. The gallery installation was a portal through which to enter a field of activity. There were scheduled video screenings of both *FTLD* and *Habit* in the museum's theater. I organized a roundtable discussion concerning treatment access issues, held in the museum's theater, involving the participation of local activists, advocates, and health care workers. The backside of the poster had a text I wrote for the exhibition, entitled "The Effort to Survive AIDS Considered from the Point of View of a Race-Car Driver." The poster was displayed around Chicago in restaurants, bars, and bookstores. A version was distributed throughout the city's bus and subway system.

The Chicago premiere of *Habit* was the centerpiece of the MCA exhibition. It was held as a benefit for the AIDS Legal Council of Chicago (ALCC), a group that provides pro bono legal services to indigent PWAs. Organizing the premiere as a benefit served a number of purposes. It raised a modest sum of money for the ALCC. I requested that the museum find donors to pay for a block of tickets so clients of the ALCC could attend, which they did. Most important, the benefit gave the ALCC much-needed publicity and visibility. The press leading up to the event included information about their efforts. I benefited greatly, too. The ALCC drew on its constituency for the event. As a result, the sold-out house at the premiere had a very diverse crowd along lines of race, gender, and class. Many people who came were not involved in any way with the art world. The screening was immediately followed by a public conversation between Douglas Crimp and me. *FTLD* and *Habit* each screened three additional times throughout the exhibition. I attended every screening to take questions.

"Drive" was a campaign to stimulate public conversation about AIDS issues, in particular the issue of access to treatment. It was very successful. The events organized for the show were well attended. The posters were everywhere. Both the *Chicago Tribune* and the *Sun Times* wrote articles about the show. I was invited to speak on the local radio. Interestingly, all the press coverage was framed as news, human interest, or public affairs. The art press didn't touch the show. Or perhaps, it didn't touch them.

The exhibition was manifold. It took on many forms: a gallery installation, video screenings, public forums, and a public poster project. When the curator, Michael Rooks, initially requested that I submit a proposal for the show, he invited me to do a video installation. I have nothing against video installations per se. However, my videos are essays. They require a setting in which the viewer can sit for extended durations. The individual parts are activated by their interrelatedness to each other. Sections of a tape can be appreciated on their own, but the work itself doesn't yield the conclusions I intend without the viewer comprehending all the parts as a whole unit. Putting my videos on a loop and projecting them continuously in a darkened room undermines the structural integrity of the work. They're intended for screenings or broadcasts, not brief encounters in galleries. So I came up with an alternative proposal. I just moved in and tried to take over as much of the museum and its resources as I could. The current context of exhibition demands that the contemporary work of art be conceptual, manifold and tactical. Within the space of a single show, the artist must work on a number of activities at once, in ways both sculptural and symphonic. In the context of my museum campaign, the substance of the work of art consists in the accrual of gestures made across the institution at every level of its functioning.

The last issue to consider regarding *Drive* is sponsorship. The pharmaceutical company Abbott Laboratories sponsored the exhibition. Abbott makes HIV medications among other medicines helpful to people with AIDS. When Michael Rooks asked me to submit a proposal for a show, it was understood that the final decision was dependent on Abbott's approval. Rooks decided to go with my proposal, but he warned me that a major drug company might not be inclined to support a show that criticized drug companies. One morning, dressed in a suit and tie, I got in a car with Michael and couple of other people from the development department of the museum, and drove to Abbott Park in a suburb of Chicago for a meeting. Although we weren't hopeful about the outcome, we poured our hearts into the presentation. I showed clips from the videos and gave copies to the press agent to show to her superiors. I told them all about the race-car and the decals, which included Abbott's logo. I shared my concepts for the public forum and the posters. They accepted it all. We were shocked.

The meeting at Abbott was instructive. The representatives of the drug company were racially diverse. There was gender parity in the room. The woman who ran the meeting was African-American. We talked a little after the meeting. She told me that she was recently hired after years of working in nonprofit AIDS organizations. The job at Abbott was an opportunity to positively influence the work of a major player in the pharmaceutical industry. The meeting confirmed what I long suspected: the image of a group of cigar-chomping white guys in a boardroom making all the decisions is not a useful, or accurate, picture of capitalism. Although the bottom line of drug companies is profit, not everyone working for them is evil. Most people care. One job of activism is to recognize the consciences of people working in the institutions we're trying to change. If you're going to wait for the revolution until you do something, you'll be waiting a long time: nothing will get done. There's an ethical principle at stake here. Don't confuse people with institutions. The illusion that individuals are identical with the institutions they work for is an institutional effect.

After the Abbott meeting, I descended into a depression and wondered if doing the show was a compromise of my ethics. In retrospect, it made sense that Abbott would support the show. It was good publicity for the company: Look how tolerant they could be! I called many of my friends, many longtime AIDS activists. All of them strongly encouraged me to do the show. Activists are used to denouncing drug companies among people who agree. This was an opportunity to do it with the opposition "in the room." It was better to inhabit a gray area than to seek the comfort of a pure position by refusing the show. I agreed to do the show under the condition that I had complete control of the project. Tensions with Abbott did arise during the exhibition, but Michael Rooks possesses unimpeachable integrity. Nothing was compromised.[19]

The sport of racing was a perfect metaphor for the issues of sponsorship played out in the exhibition. First, my effort to survive is underwritten much like the way race-car drivers are sponsored. I take twenty pills a day, all made by major drug companies, to stay alive. Car racing is as

19. The budget for my MCA show was fifteen thousand dollars. Every penny was spent on the show through the agency of the museum.

much about the sponsors as it is about the skill of the driver and the expertise of his crew. The team with the most resources usually wins. Second, the exhibition itself was underwritten by corporate sponsorship; many museum shows are in some part sponsored by corporate donations.

A closing image: the racetrack is elliptical. Cars go around and around, the same drivers compete in different tournaments, occasionally there are huge pile-ups. The outcome is never certain.

[Teaching]

We are not feeling the same thing and
We are not feeling it at the same time.[20]

A preoccupation with problems of education is evident in all of my work. In the essay "Geography Notes," I contemplated Andrea Fraser's docent activity as a model practice. Throughout the eighties and early nineties, I made AIDS education full-time. For the past decade of experimental film and video production a commitment to pedagogy has linked all of my activities. The imperative to educate people about AIDS is a consistent feature of my efforts. The production of knowledge is another recurring concern. Two questions continue to shape my all of my research: How do we come to know what we know? How do we come to believe what we know is true?

There is nowhere more challenging to theories of pedagogy than the classroom. I teach. From my earliest formulation of practice, I understood

20. Bertolt Brecht, "The Moment Before Impact," *Bertolt Brecht Poems 1913–1956*, eds. John Willet and Ralph Manheim (London and New York: Methuen, 1979), p. 342.

that teaching had to play a role. All the artists I admired taught or lectured. I began working in classrooms toward the end of the eighties.

Bertolt Brecht's practice is the origin of an instructive model of production that joins education to popular entertainment. In the lines quoted above, Brecht considers how an actor and an audience coincide in time and space. Both are present in the same space, at the same moment, and though they follow different trajectories they are united around the same action.

The Brechtian theater actor and the classroom teacher perform similarly. The job of the teacher is much more than imparting information and facts. Education is only partly practical. The most important contribution a teacher can make is to magnetize knowledge itself, to electrify the classroom in ways that animate the act of learning with a sense of purpose, and most important, joy.

In 1997, I applied for my first full-time teaching job. The application required that I provide a philosophy of teaching. This is what I submitted.

1.0 Teaching is the art of learning.

1.1 Learning is the acquisition of methods.

1.2 Methods are the means to solve problems.

2.0 The teacher's method is the art of the question.

2.1 A question is a burden.

2.2 Learning is a process of overcoming a series of increasingly difficult burdens.

3.0 Teaching is an act of devotion.

3.1 A teacher must never abandon students to the harsh difficulties of learning.

3.2 The teacher shares the burdens of learning with the students.

4.0 Learning is both painful and enjoyable.

4.1 The teacher must protect students from undue pain and undue enjoyment.

4.2 Learning is neither a cruel exercise nor a crude entertainment.

5.0 Learning is the joining of ideas to actions.

5.1 The teacher teaches that every action is the cause of an idea.

5.2 The teacher provides neither the idea nor the action.

5.3 The teacher provides the mediation between the idea and the action.

6.0 The teacher teaches learning.

6.1 Learning teaches the students.

6.2 Learning teaches the teacher to teach.

[Reading and Writing]

I urge my students to read, advocating a wide range of writing: fiction, poetry, philosophy, and critical theory. Reading has been the primary vehicle for my own intellectual activity. Written language, the grammar of sentences, the choice of words, punctuation, and verb tense, all of it together is the filter system through which knowledge flows. Like a Greek philosopher reducing the world to the qualities of one element, such as fire or water, I am tempted to state that all is writing.

My disposition toward the written word has its origins in my own religious education. I read the Torah, and though I am a secular intellectual, I genuinely believe that it contains the world. The Old Testament contains all the ugly primitive feelings known to humankind. It also contains the loftiest aspirations. The ideals expressed in the Torah would mean nothing without the petty, hateful opinions and actions written within the text. Many people reject the Bible for its prejudices. The injunction against homosexuality is one example of its childish and phobic formulations. The detailed descriptions of animal sacrifice and communal slaughter are abhorrent. Even God is spiteful, angry, and capricious. These negative qualities are the elements worthy of contemplation in the Bible. The Torah presents a history of bad behavior by people who are trying their best to be good. Stonings and shunnings, the attribution of blame in every direction, the relentless guilt—all that's recorded in the Torah is massively instructive about the misuse of faith. And yet, I have faith. I have faith in the capacity of writing to amplify the reader's ability to think and act for the better.

Texts can change the reader's body. They alter the affects, produce unfamiliar sensations, and open up the mind to novelty. These are not merely mental alterations; they are physiological changes. Making art demands a kind of athleticism. I can't imagine any more effective kind of training to advance one's practice than a rigorous bibliography. I don't have a specific reading list in mind. Each artist is responsible for their own criteria.

Speculative thought is the engine of art production. Art is the proving ground of ideas. It should never merely illustrate concepts. And artists do more than read theory. Many theorize their own practices. The blank page is the perfect laboratory environment to assess one's production. Of course, it is no replacement for practice. It's part of the practice. Historical conditions necessitated that I incorporate theoretical reflections of my own output into my work. The conditions are twofold. First, the dissolution of medium-specificity and the resultant diversification of artist's labor in the sixties elevated the status of the artist's writing to the level of other kinds of art making. Second, the AIDS crisis required a tactical mode of practice, achieving competence in many fields.

[Conclusion: Return to Figure A.]

The schema drawn at the beginning of this essay locates the camera at the center of its order. The location of the camera in the diagram is analogous to the position of the subject in the order of consciousness. The front, the back, the inside and the outside—these are the coordinates of the body. The angle of your perceptions, your shifting point of view—they're both affected by light and speed. Every day the sun returns, you wake up, and the world makes another complete revolution. You spend your days awake and your nights asleep. Still, the conscious and the unconscious processes of your mind get confused: you often dream on the job and sometimes you run in your sleep.

What goes on in your mind is only partially observable to others. We all have secrets; the best we even keep from ourselves. Why shouldn't we lock some of ourselves up and hide the key? Everyone's watching. The audience applauds you even when you're alone. Take comfort. Relax. There is not one member of the audience, living or dead, who has any conclusive interpretation of the meaning of your secrets.

The time-concept in figure A. is an abstraction. The units of measure we use to mark time are mere conventions. There is no standard other than human invention guaranteeing the movement of a clock's hands. I don't have evidence to support this, but I suspect that the origin of the ticking clock is the body's heartbeat. I don't think about my heart much. I'm only aware of it beating when I climb stairs too fast; or when I'm startled. I take the heart for granted like I do all of my organs. I don't pay attention until attention is demanded. I treat my wristwatch the same way, consulting it only after I've lost track of time or some appointment demands my attention.

The perception of time changes with circumstance. I spent nearly half of my life assuming that I'd die in the near future. Now, with the help of new medications it seems possible that I may live a "normal" life span. Though my health is good at the moment, my fear of death was compounded by this project. Writing the concluding essay felt like writing my own epitaph. Now it's done and no more words come to mind. There are plenty of ideas, but none yet coalesce into a form I can share. New theoretical frameworks now emerging, new directions to take, and projects to make, they will all have to wait for another time. That there will be another time is a remarkable conjecture. When this book appears I will have turned forty. Imagine that. I can't. And yet, here it is.

VIDEO/FILMOGRAPHY

Portraits of AIDS Care Providers and Advocates, six separate works each approximately six minutes, produced, directed and edited for the AIDS Legal Council of Chicago, digital video, 2002

Habit, produced directed, edited, 52 minutes, digital video, 2001

Treatment Action Campaign, produced, directed, edited, 10 minutes, digital video, 2000

The Suicide, director, editor, screenplay adaptation; 88 minutes, 16mm, Beta-SP, 1996

A Cloud in Trousers, director, editor; 31 minutes, 16mm, Beta-SP, 1995

Fast Trip, Long Drop, producer, director, writer; 56 minutes, 16mm, Beta-SP, 1993

Portraits of People Living With HIV #1–#9, producer, director, camera, editor, 2–10 minutes each, video, 1992–1995

It is what it is . . . , producer, director, editor, 58 minutes, video, 1992

Living with AIDS—Gay Men's Health Crisis weekly cable television show. Broadcast twice a week on Manhattan, Brooklyn, Queens, and Staten Island Public Access. Produced by Gregg Bordowitz and Jean Carlomusto, including:

- "Thinking About Death," coproducer, codirector, 28 minutes, 1991
- "An Informed Approach to HIV Testing," coproducer, codirector, 28 minutes, 1990
- "Living Proof," coproducer, codirector, 25 minutes, 1990
- "Safer-Sex Shorts," coproducer, codirector, 25 minutes, 1990
- "Seize Control of the FDA," coproducer, codirector, 29 minutes, 1989
- "PWA Power: Life after Diagnosis," coproducer, codirector, 29 minutes, 1989

["Work Your Body: Options for People Who Are HIV Antibody Positive," coproducer, codirector, 28 minutes, 1988

DIVA TV—Damned Interfering Video Activists, a collective of AIDS Activists, founding member.

Pride, 28 minutes, 1989

. . . some aspect of a shared lifestyle . . . producer, writer, and director, 20 minutes, video, 1986

Target City Hall, 28 minutes, 1989

Testing the Limits Collective, collective of lesbians, gays, and straights formed in 1987 to document AIDS activism, founding member

Testing the Limits: New York City, coproducer, codirector, co-editor, 30 minutes, video, 1988

SELECTED WRITINGS OF GREGG BORDOWITZ

"Mapping Georgia On My Mind." Gallery statement in exhibition catalog, Thirty-Third Atlanta Arts Festival, September 20–28, 1986, Piedmont Park Visual Arts Division, pp. 38–39.

"Geography Notes: A Survey." *Real Life Magazine,* no. 16 (autumn 1986): 12–17.

"Picture a Coalition." *October* 43 (winter 1987): 183–196.

"Picture a Coalition." In *AIDS: Cultural Analysis Cultural Activism,* edited by Douglas Crimp, pp. 183–196. Cambridge, Massachusetts, and London: The MIT Press, 1988.

"Sex, Sexuality, Eroticism, and Desire." *The Guardian: Independent Radical Newsweekly,* September 21, 1988, p. 20.

"Art and Activism: A Conversation between Douglas Crimp and Gregg Bordowitz." In catalog from the conference "AIDS: The Artist's Response," held February 24–April 16, 1989, at the Hoyt L. Sherman Gallery of The Ohio State University.

"Who Is Art." *Outweek* (October 22, 1989): 57, 63.

"Experiments in Gay Filmmaking." *The Guardian: Independent Radical Newsweekly,* September 13 1989, p. 24.

"Revenge of the Teenage Perverts." *The Guardian: Independent Radical Newsweekly,* July 17, 1991, p. 20.

"Against Heterosexuality." *Parkett* 27 (1991): 100–104.

"Identity Crisis: Queer Politics in the Age of Possibilities. A Conversation with Marcellus Blount, Gregg Bordowitz, Holly Hughes, Jeff Nunokowa, Eve Sedgewick, Alisa Solomon." *Village Voice,* June 30, 1992, pp. 27–29, 33.

"By All Means Possible." *Village Voice,* July 28, 1992, pp. 36, 41.

"Do It! Safer Sex for Boys and Girls Comes of Age." Cowritten with Jean Carlomusto. In *A Leap In The Dark: AIDS, Art, and Contemporary Cultures,* edited by Allan Klusacek and Ken Morrison, pp. 177–183. Montreal: Vehicle Press, 1992.

"The AIDS Crisis Is Ridiculous." In *Queer Looks,* edited by Martha Gever, John Greyson, and Prahtiba Parmar, pp. 208–224. London and New York: Routledge, 1993.

"Boat Trip." *American Imago* (Johns Hopkins University) 51, no. 1 (spring 1994): 105–125.

"Dense Moments without Reason." In *Uncontrollable Bodies,* edited by Rodney Sappington and Tyler Stawlings, pp. 25–43. Seattle: Bay Press, 1994.

"*Schindler's List/Philadelphia.*" *Frieze International Art Magazine,* no. 15 (March-April 1994): 54–55.

"The AIDS Crisis Is Not Over: A Conversation with Gregg Bordowitz, Douglas Crimp, and Laura Pinsky," by Cathy Caruth and Thomas Keenan. In *Trauma: Explorations in Memory,* edited and with an introduction by Cathy Caruth, pp. 256–271. Baltimore and London: Johns Hopkins University Press, 1995.

"Double Dare: Interview with Gregg Bordowitz and Isaac Julien," by Abby Nolan. *Village Voice,* vol. 40, January 10, 1995.

"Art of Living: James Meyer talks with Gregg Bordowitz." *Artforum* 33, no. 10 (summer 1995): 89–90, 128.

"Operative Assumptions." In *Resolutions: Contemporary Video Practices,* edited by Michael Renov and Erika Suderburg, pp. 173–184. Minneapolis and London: University of Minnesota Press, 1996.

"Present Tense." In *Processed Lives: Gender and Technology in Everyday Life,* edited by Jennifer Terry and Melodie Calvert, pp. 104–105. London and New York: Routledge, 1997.

"Guest List For A Cocktail Party." *Camerawork* 25, no. 1 (spring/summer 1998): 4–9.

"Fast Trip, Long View: Talking to Gregg Bordowitz." Interview with Robert Atkins, in *Artery: The AIDS-Arts Journal,* an online journal available at <http://www.artistswithaids.org/artery/index1.html>, 2000.

"What Is More Important: The Word or the Idea?" In *Bodies of Resistance,* exhibition catalog for "Visual AIDS and Real Art Ways," Connecticut, 2000.

"New York Was Yesterday." Ongoing column in *Documents: A Magazine of Contemporary Art and Visual Culture,* nos. 7–16 (1996–2000).

"The Drug User." Text written for a gallery show entitled "Something Happened," curated by Sally Berger at Apex Art Curatorial Program, New York, November 2000.

"Network Society." *Art Journal,* four installments (winter 2000, spring 2001, summer 2001, fall 2001).

"Drive: The AIDS Crisis Is Still Beginning." A collection of essays, dialogues, and texts surrounding Gregg Bordowitz's films *Fast Trip, Long Drop* and *Habi*t, and his exhibition *Drive,* held at the Museum of Contemporary Art Chicago, April 6–July 7, 2002. Contributors: Douglas Crimp, Bill Horrigan, Yvonne, Ranier, Michael Rooks, Kendall Thoomas, Lynne Tillman, Gregg Bordowitz. In *White Walls* journal, edited by Anthony Elms (fall 2002).

"Force of Habit." Unpublished interview by Richard Morrison, 2003.

"My Postmodernism." *Artforum* 41, no. 7 (March 2003): 226–229, 273–274.

"An Interview with the 12th Session of the Ecole Du Magasin," and "A Conversation with Gregg Bordowitz," by Amely Greeven and Stephen Sprot. In *AIDS Riot New York 1987–1994: Artist Collectives Against AIDS,* pp. 217–220, 307–310. France: Magasin, 2003.

"Dawn's Early Light." In *Image Stream,* catalog edited by Helen Molesworth, Wexner Center for the Arts, The Ohio State University, pp. 76–83. Columbus, Ohio, 2003.

INDEX

The MIT Press Writing Art series
edited by Roger Conover

Art After Philosophy and After: Collected Writings, 1966–1990
by Joseph Kosuth

Rock My Religion: Writings and Projects 1965–1990
by Dan Graham

Continuous Project Altered Daily: The Writings of Robert Morris (OCTOBER)
by Robert Morris

Remote Control: Power, Cultures, and the World of Appearances
by Barbara Kruger

The Daily Practice of Painting: Writings 1960–1993
by Gerhard Richter

Reasons for Knocking at an Empty House: Writings 1973–1994
by Bill Viola

Out of Order, Out of Sight—Vol. I: Selected Writings in Meta-Art 1968–1992
by Adrian Piper

Out of Order, Out of Sight—Vol. II: Selected Writings in Art Criticism 1967–1992
by Adrian Piper

Imaging Desire
by Mary Kelly

Destruction of the Father/Reconstruction of the Father: Writings and Interviews, 1923–1997
by Louise Bourgeois

Critical Vehicles: Writings, Projects, Interviews
by Krzysztof Wodiczko

Two-Way Mirror Power: Selected Writings by Dan Graham on His Art
by Dan Graham

Imaging Her Erotics: Essays, Interviews, Projects
by Carolee Schneemann

Essays on Art and Language
by Charles Harrison

Conceptual Art and Painting: Further Essays on Art and Language
by Charles Harrison

Leave Any Information at the Signal: Writings, Interviews, Bits, Pages (OCTOBER)
by Ed Ruscha

Foul Perfection: Essays and Criticism
by Mike Kelley

Please Pay Attention Please: Bruce Nauman's Words: Writings and Interviews
by Bruce Nauman

Decoys and Disruptions: Selected Writings, 1975–2001 (OCTOBER)
by Martha Rosler

Minor Histories: Statements, Conversations, Proposals
by Mike Kelley

The AIDS Crisis Is Ridiculous and Other Writings, 1986–2003
by Gregg Bordowitz

Printed by Libri Plureos GmbH in Hamburg,
Germany

9 780262 524599